THE SIRT
DIET

The Ultimate Guide to Lose 7lbs In Just 7 days Activating Your Skinny Gene with Sirt Foods, Over 100 Top, Easy and Delicious Recipes.

Table of Contents

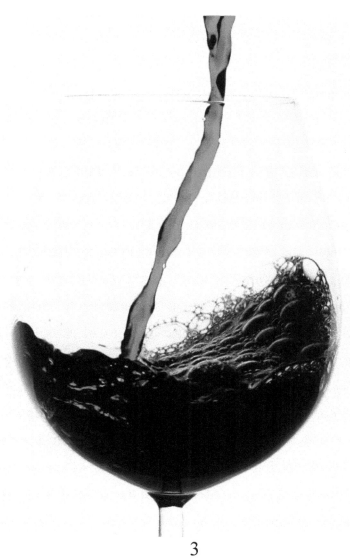

3

Introduction

Explore the initial experience of a foreign diet— that will help you lose seven pounds in seven days while enjoying enduring vitality and consuming all the foods you enjoy. Fasting has become a popular diet choice during the last few years. The Sirtfood Diet plan focuses on upping the balanced sirtfood intake. These include oranges, citrus fruits, parsley, capers, blueberries, green tea, corn, strawberries, turmeric, olive oil, red onion, rocket, and that beloved kale of the old health-lover.

The diet-eating plan for Sirtfood is focused on polyphenols, natural compounds found in plant foods that help protect the body's cells from inflammation or death from the disease. A small group of polyphenols will imitate the effects of diet and exercise by triggering the body's sirtuin, also known as "skinny" genes, according to fitness experts Aidan Goggins and Glen Matten, who invented the Sirtfood Diet.

The SIRT diet helps you to eat chocolate and drink red wine, so no doubt it's the 2020 trend in wellness. So if you've tried and failed a healthy diet program, this book could be the ideal option for a happy, safer you if it includes the SIRT lifestyle program. It also contains chocolate and red wine, so that we're always finished. If you embark on a healthy eating regime, candy and alcohol are usually the first things to go, but the opposite is true of the Sirtfood diet plan. Nutrition experts behind the diet say that you can' turn on the fat-burning forces of your body' by eating foods rich in a type of protein called sirtuin activators. Two foods high inactivators of the sirtuin are Dark Chocolate and Red Wine.

Who came up with the Sirtfood Diet?

A group of writers and fitness experts named Aidan Goggins and Glen Matten, who always has focused on eating healthy rather than weight loss.

Why is the Sirtfood diet good news?

Unlike other diet plans specifically geared to dramatic and unhealthy weight loss, the Sirtfood diet is perfect if you just want to boost your immune system, pack in some vitamins, and feel a little healthier.

The sirtuin activators will help regulate your metabolism, increase your muscle, and burn fat as well as help you feel energized.

The objective of the Sirt diet is more about healthy eating than dramatic weight loss, but some nutritionists have taken leaving out to the fact that their book is decorated with the "lose 7lbs in 7 days" tag line. A reduction of 1 to 2lbs a week is considered a stable and safe number. So much dramatic weight loss may not be ideal for your well-being in a short time. Also, obvious but relevant: red wine is full of toxins, even if it is high in sirtuin activators, so it probably isn't a good idea to guzzle it as part of a' diet.'

In recent years, the Sirtfood diet has become just as popular as the Cabbage Soup Diet, the 5.2 diets, and the Dukan Diet. But is it yet another diet that pledges too much, or can it help you slim down and feel better adopting a sirtfood eating plan?

We've distinguished fact from fiction to show you everything about the Sirtfood Diet you need to know. Read on to find out all you need to know about the SIRT diet is perfect for you.

Chapter 1

Sirtfood

"Sirtfood" sounds like something created by humans, bringing to earth in the hopes of gaining the power of the mind and world domination for human consumption. Sirtfoods are simply foods rich in sirtuins.

Sirtuins are a type of protein that has been shown to control metabolism, increase muscle mass, and burn fat by experiments on fruit flies and mice.

A' set meal' is a food that is rich in sirtuin activators. Again, sirtuins are a kind of protein that prevents the cells in our bodies from dying or becoming inflamed by illness. Still, testing has also shown that they can help regulate the metabolism, improve muscle, and burn fat-hence the current' wonder food' name.

Sirtfoods are foods high in sirtuin protein, which is a form of plant-based protein that has shown some potential to improve metabolic health in clinical studies. Sirt grocery includes:

Medjool dates

Blueberries

Coffee

Kale

Arugula

Parsley

Celery

Green apple

Soy

Strawberries

85 percent cocoa chocolate

Turmeric

This program will help you burn fat and improve your strength by using the sirtfood, priming your body for long-term weight loss success and a longer, safer, illness-free life. All this while they drink red wine. It sounds like the perfect meal.

How does it work?

The secret to weight loss is quite easy at its core: either build a calorie deficit by increasing your calorie consumption by exercise or decrease your calorie intake. But what if you can skip the diet and activate a "skinny gene" without the need for an intense calorie restriction instead? That is The Sirtfood Diet's idea. The way to do that is through sirtfoods.

Sirt foods are rich in nutrients that cause a sirtuin called a so-called "skinny gene." The "skinny gene" is triggered when an energy deficit is produced after the calories are limited. In 2003, sirtuins became important to the field of nutrition when researchers found that resveratrol, a compound form in red wine, had the same impact on life expectancy as calorie restriction but was accomplished without restricting consumption. In the 2015 pilot analysis (conducted by Goggins and Matten) investigating the potency of sirtuins, the 39 subjects lost an average of seven pounds in seven days. Those findings sound impressive, but understanding this is a small sample size analyzed over a short time is important. Weight-loss critics have concerns about the lofty promises, too. "The claims made are very theoretical and extrapolate from studies that focused mostly on simple organisms (such as yeast) at the cellular level. What occurs at the cellular level does not necessarily translate into what happens at the macro level in the human body," says Adrienne Youdim, M.D., Center for Weight Loss and Nutrition at Beverly Hills, CA.

What kind of foods are high in sirtuins?

Foods high in sirtuins, which looks more like a compilation of trendy ingredients than a complex new diet. Examples include arugula, chilies, chocolate, green tea, Medjool dates, red wine, turmeric, walnuts, and the favorite-kale health-conscious. While the diet that is being marketed as safe, it will not automatically encourage weight loss on its own.

Which does the diet entail?

The diet is given in two stages. Phase 1 lasts three days and reduces calories to 1,000 per day, consisting of three green juices and a meal

9

approved for sirtfood. Phase two lasts four days and increases the daily allotment by two green juices and two meals to 1,500 calories per day.

There is a nutrition program after these stages that is not based on calories but on small servings, well-balanced meals, and filling up on mainly sirt foods. The 14-day maintenance plan includes three dinners, one green juice, and one or two snacks with sirtfood bits. Followers are also inspired to complete 30 minutes of activity five days a week per recommendation from the government, but it is not the plan's main focus.

The Sirtfood diet consists of two phases; the first lasts a week, and the second lasts two weeks. You're limited to 1,000 calories from one sirtfood meal and three green juices during the first three days of the plan. You can consume two sirtfood meals and two green juices per day for the rest of the first week. The daily meal schedule for step two consists of three sirtfoods and green juice.

The Asian Shrimp Stir-Fry with Buckwheat Noodles and Strawberry Buckwheat Tabbouleh have nutritious, sirtfood-rich meals. Continue to include sirtfoods in your meals to continue getting effects beyond the initial three-week "jumpstart" span.

If you are not deviating from the schedule, the Sirtfood Diet guarantees a weight loss of seven pounds in the first week (without losing muscle mass). "It also appears to have anti-aging benefits, to help improve the regulation of memory and blood sugar, and to reduce chronic disease risk."

What can you eat on the Sirtfood Diet?

The headline-grabbers for the Sirtfood Diet are red wine and dark chocolate because both appear to be rich in sirtuin activators. Though, that's not the whole picture, and you're not going to feel the effects of mainlining Merlot and Green & Blacks.

The Sirtfood Diet plan focuses on upping the balanced sirtfood intake. These include oranges, citrus fruits, parsley, capers, blueberries, green tea, corn, strawberries, turmeric, olive oil, red onion, rocket, and that beloved kale of the old health-lover.

Ironically, coffee is another top sirtfood, which is welcome news if you're fed up being told to cut caffeine. Countries where people already eat a vast amount of sirt foods include Japan and Italy, both of which are regularly ranked among the healthiest countries in the world.

Most of the ingredients can be found easily and are well known as healthy choices. Yet additional ingredients, including lovage, buckwheat, and matcha green tea powder, may be harder to find.

"What can't you eat?

Officially, no foods on the Sirtfood Diet are "banned," but the calorie restriction is severe — especially during the initial three days when you're limited to 1,000 calories. To put that in perspective, according to the USDA Dietary Guidelines for 2015-2020, 1000 calories is the recommended intake for a sedentary 2-to 3-year-old.

Is there a Sirtfood Diet plan?

Yes, it is! You limit your intake to 1000 calories per day for the first week, which includes consuming three sirtfood green juices and one sirtfood rich meal a day. You increase your diet to 1500 calories a day the next week and eat two sirt-rich meals and two natural juices. However, there's no set plan, in the long run, it's all about adjusting your lifestyle to include as many sirt foods as you can, which should make you feel healthier and more energized. For more details, please see point 5 (below).

What are the benefits?

If you follow that diet closely, you will lose weight. "If you consume 1,000 calories of tacos, 1,000 calories of spinach, or 1,000 calories of snickerdoodles, you'll lose weight at 1,000 calories! But she also pointed out that you can achieve with a more realistic calorie restriction. The average daily calorie intake of someone not on a diet is 2,000 to 2,200, and lowering to 1,500 is still moderate and would be an efficient weight-loss. Losing muscle is synonymous with lowering the metabolic rate or' metabolism,' which makes it more difficult to maintain weight.

Are there any precaution

There are other methods you can minimize your calorie intake without being so limited in the food you eat. That being said, the diet isn't necessarily "unhealthy," so if a woman found success, she wouldn't automatically be wary against it.

When you follow this program, make sure to eat plenty of nutrients and change the food you eat to minimize shortages in vitamins. Want you to want? The diet is incredibly strict and has not been properly proven to be effective. You are much better off cultivating a diet in the amounts that fit the individual needs to consume a range of whole foods.

The Sirtfood Diet guarantees weight and fat reduction without a lack of muscle focused on eating a certain set of balanced, polyphenol-rich foods.

Are there any drawbacks?

The hardest part of the Sirtfood Diet is calorie restriction and reliance on green juice, and this may be unhealthy for some groups of people. I wouldn't prescribe this diet to patients with certain drugs, such as Coumadin, or health conditions such as diabetes. Even if you're in extensive training or are pregnant or breastfeeding, she should give it a miss.

"I don't generally recommend any diets that depend on unnecessarily stringent external laws. "Nevertheless, many of the recommended' sirtfoods' promote health, and I would recommend that people incorporate these into their meals. As always, I strongly inspire people to listen to the appetite and satiety signals in their bodies for advice on when and how much food to eat. "This approach is questionable in terms of long-term survival. Once you've been through the first few weeks, there's no diet plan to implement but to add more Sirtfoods to each meal. It makes the diet much more forgiving than most, which is an enormous benefit. Still, a starvation period of three weeks could easily lead to overeating during phase two, eventually putting you back to square one.

This is still a difficult diet to follow, even if you're uber-disciplined. "A mere 1,000 calories will leave most people feeling very thirsty. However, if you're not a lover of green juice, a favorite of the first week, it will make you even more hungry," she says. Additionally, since most of the weight loss in step one is water weight, it will return as soon as you start eating normally.

Science of Sirtuin

Sirtuins help to control cell safety. They focus on NAD+ to work. Sirtuins are a protein family that regulates cellular health. Sirtuins are instrumental in regulating cellular homeostasis. Homeostasis means that the cell is kept in balance. However, sirtuins can only react in the presence of the NAD+, a coenzyme found in all living cells, nicotinamide adenine dinucleotide.

How Sirtuins Regulate Cellular Health with NAD+

Think of the cells in your body as a workplace. There are many employees in the workplace working on different projects with the ultimate goal: to remain competitive and to accomplish the company's purpose efficiently for as long as possible. There are also many parts in the cells working on different activities with one ultimate goal: stay healthy and run properly for as long as possible. Just as business priorities change because of different internal and external causes, so do cell priorities. Someone has to manage the workplace, overseeing

15

where, who'll do it, and when to turn direction. That would be your CEO in the office. They're the sirtuins in the body at the cellular level. Sirtuins are kin of seven proteins that have a part to play in cell protection. The sirtuins can only act in the presence of NAD+, a coenzyme present in all living cells, nicotinamide adenine dinucleotide. NAD+ is essential to cellular metabolism and hundreds of other processes in biology. If sirtuins are the CEO of a company, then NAD+ is the money that pays the CEO and workers ' salaries, all while keeping the lights on and the rent paid for office space. Without it, a business, and the body, cannot work. Yet NAD+ levels decline with age, reducing sirtuin activity also with age. It's not that easy, as all of the stuff in the human body. Sirtuins are managing whatever happens in your cells.

Sirtuins are proteins. What does that mean?

The sirtuins are a protein family. Protein that sounds like dietary protein— what's contained in beans and vegetables, and well, protein shakes — but in this condition, we're talking about molecules called proteins that act in some different roles throughout the body's cells. Think of proteins as a company's teams, each focussing on their specific function when collaborating with other divisions.

A well-known protein in the body system is hemoglobin, which is a part of the protein globin family and is responsible for carrying

16

oxygen throughout your blood. The myoglobin is the counterpart of the hemoglobin, and together they form the family of globins.

Your body has almost 60,000 protein families-many departments! — And the sirtuins are a family of these. While hemoglobin is one in a two-protein family, sirtuins are a 7-fold family.

Of the cell's seven sirtuins, three work in the mitochondria, three work in the nucleus, and one works in the cytoplasm, each playing a variety for functions. However, the fundamental role of sirtuins is to remove the acetyl groups from other proteins.

Acetyl groups regulate the basic reactions. They're actual protein tags known by other proteins that will communicate with them. If proteins are the cell departments, and DNA is the CEO, each department head's availability status is for the acetyl groups. For example, if a protein is available, then the sirtuin can work with it to make something happen, just as the CEO can work with a department head available to get something happening.

Sirtuins function with classes of acetyls by doing what is called deacetylation. This means they know that on a molecule, there is an acetyl group and eliminate the acetyl group, which is teeing up the molecule for their work. One way sirtuins function is by eliminating biological proteins, such as histones, from the acetyl groups (deacetylating). Sirtuins, for example, deacetylate histones, proteins that form part of a condensed form of DNA called chromatin. The

17

histone is a big, voluminous protein around which the DNA coils itself. Speak of it as a Christmas tree, and the ocean with DNA is the island with decorations. The chromatin is free or unwound when the histones have an acetyl ring.

This unwound chromatin means the transcription of the DNA, which is an essential process. But it doesn't need to remain unwound, as in this position it's vulnerable to damage, almost like the Christmas lights could get tangled or the bulbs could get damaged when they're unwieldy or too long up. The chromatin is locked or firmly and conveniently damaged when the histones are deacetylated by sirtuins, meaning gene expression is interrupted or silenced.

The principal function of sirtuins was discovered in the 1990s. Researchers have flocked to study them since then, identifying their significance while also raising questions about what else we can learn about it.

Sirtuin activating compound.

Given their beneficial effects in fostering survival, proteins from the sirtuin family are a very promising target for medications. Sirtuin-activating compounds (STACs), including plant-copied metabolites and the well-known resveratrol, are the first and most active sirtuin activator and have been shown to longer life span in various species. Synthetic activators like SRT1720 and SRT2104 improve the metabolic profile and extend mice's lifespan and healthspan under a high-fat, normal diet. Interestingly, SRT1720 improves insulin sensitivity, lowers plasma glucose, and increases mitochondrial capacity in models of experimental diabetes, representing a promising new therapeutic approach to the treatment of age-related diseases such as type 2 diabetes;

Besides, resveratrol exerts anti-inflammatory effects in visceral white adipose tissue in rhesus monkeys, under a high-fat and high-sugar diet. Resveratrol defends against the symptoms of obesity, and age-related metabolic loss in mice and nonhuman primates fed a high-fat diet, increases insulin sensitivity and mitochondrial functions, and inhibits hepatic steatosis.

Resveratrol additionally delays the onset of neurodegeneration and improves learning and memory in aged mice. The promising results in preclinical models have prompted the physicians to study resveratrol in humans where it has beneficial effects on the aged and the obese. Resveratrol also has positive effects on systolic blood pressure, hemoglobin A1c and creatinine in people with type 2 diabetes. Synthetic STACS also has been shown to have positive cardiovascular effects on active smoking with tobacco.

The mechanism behind resveratrol's beneficial effects is unclear as it has been proposed that resveratrol's direct stimulation of sirtuin 1 is an in vitro artifact and that resveratrol acts mainly by stimulating AMPK, possibly by inhibiting phosphodiesterases (PDE). AMPK can then indirectly activate sirtuin one by elevating its cosubstrate NAD+ to intracellular levels. Alternatively, resveratrol may initially activate sirtuin 1 in vivo, resulting in activation of AMPK through deacetylation and activation of the AMPK kinase LKB1.

How Sirtfood Diet Works

Sirtfood Diet is one of the most recent trendy new diets starting to crop up regularly. It has become a favorite of Europe's celebrities and is known for allowing red wine and chocolate. The founders maintain that it's not a fad, but that "sirt diets" are the key to unlocking fat loss and disease prevention. Health experts, however, warn that this diet may not live up to the hype, and may even be a bad idea.

The sirtfood diet works off the concept that by eating certain things, you can cause the activation of certain proteins called sirtuins or colloquially dubbed "skinny genes." According to Healthline, sirtuins have any capacity. They are "a group of seven proteins found in the body that have been shown to manage a variety of functions, including metabolism, inflammation, and lifespan." There are two diet-stages.

Sirtfood Diet was developed by two celebrity nutritionists working for a private gym in the U.K. We market the diet as a revolutionary new diet and health plan that works by flipping on your "skinny button." This diet is based on sirtuin science (SIRTs), a group of seven proteins found in the body that has been shown to control a variety of functions, including appetite, inflammation, and longevity. Other natural plant compounds that increase the level of these proteins in the body, and the foods containing them have been called "sirtfoods." The diet incorporates sirtfoods with calorie restriction, both of which can cause the body to produce higher sirtuin levels. The Sirtfood diet can result

21

in rapid weight loss, all while retaining muscle mass and shielding you from chronic illness. Once you've completed the diet, you're encouraged to continue your regular diet, including sirtfoods and the signature green juice of the diet.

Sirtfoods work by activating the body's so-called "skinny gene" pathways, the same genes that are activated when we are exercising or quick.

This helps the body burn fat in a way that mimics the restriction on calories but without the loss of nutrients or other deficiencies. The sample of people studying the diet, with increased muscle mass and signs of feeling full and satisfied with food intake, showed an average loss of 7 pounds of weight in 7 days.

"Sirtfoods act as a master organizer of our whole metabolism, most importantly having effects on fat burning while at the same time enlarging muscle and improving cellular activity." Through their study, Goggins and Matten found that many of the foods falling into the Stirfood group are already frequently correlated with the world's healthiest diets-like the traditional Mediterranean diet.

Is it effective?

This diet will result in super-charge weight loss, turn the "skinny gene" on, and prevent disease.

The thing is they don't have any evidence to back them up.

There is no convincing confirmation to date that the Sirtfood Diet has a more beneficial effect on weight loss than any other diet limited by calories. And although many of those foods have healthy properties, no long-term human studies have been conducted to determine whether taking a diet rich in sirtfoods has any concrete health benefits. Participants may follow the diet for one week and exercise daily. Participants will lose an average of 7 pounds (3.2 kg) at the end of the week and retain or even gain muscle mass. Yet these findings are hardly shocking. Limiting your calorie intake to 1,000 calories, and actively exercising, will almost always cause weight loss. Regardless, this kind of rapid weight loss is neither genuine nor long-lasting, and after the first week, this study did not follow participants to see if they gained any of the weight back, which is typically so.

As well as burning fat and muscle, when your body is deprived of energy, it uses its emergency energy stores or glycogen.

Each glycogen molecule requires 3–4 water molecules for storage. If the body uses glycogen, the water always gets rid of it. It is known as the "water weight." Only about one-third of the weight loss develop from fat during the first week of extreme calorie restriction, while the other two-thirds come from water, muscle, and glycogen.

Your body will replenish its glycogen stores as soon as your calorie intake increases, and the weight returns right back.

However, this form of calorie restriction can also cause your body to lower its metabolic rate, allowing energy requirements to be even lower in calories per day. This diet is likely to help you lose a few pounds in the beginning, but it'll probably return as soon as the diet is over.

As far as disease prevention is concerned, it is likely three weeks not long enough to have any measurable long-term impact. On the other side, it may very well be a smart idea to add sirtfood to your regular diet over the long term. You might as well skip the diet in that case, and start doing it now.

This diet will help you lose weight because it is low in calories, but when the diet finishes, the weight is likely to return. The diet is too brief to have an effect on your health in the long term, so you can stay in it.

Chapter 2

Blue Zones

In old age, chronic diseases are becoming increasingly common. While genetics determine your lifespan and susceptibility to these diseases somewhat, your lifestyle will likely have a more significant impact. A couple of places in the world are called "Blue Zones." The term refers to geographic areas where people have low chronic disease rates and live longer than anywhere else.

"Blue Zone" is a non-scientific term granted to geographical regions that are home to some of the oldest people in the world. They are called Blue Zones because they drew blue circles around them on a map when Buettner and his associate were searching for these areas. Five known blue zones:

Icaria (Greece): Icaria is an island in Greece where human beings eat a nutritious Mediterranean diet of olive oil, red wine, and organic vegetables.

Ogliastra, Sardinia (Italy): Some of the world's oldest people live in the region of Ogliastra, Sardinia. They live in the mountainous areas where, typically, they work on farms and drink lots of red wine.

Okinawa (Japan): Okinawa is home to the oldest women in the world who eat plenty of soy-based food and perform tai chi, a form of meditative exercise.

Nicoya Peninsula (Costa Rica): The Nicoya diet is based on corn tortillas and beans. The people in this area regularly perform physical jobs into old age and have a life purpose known as "plan de Vida."

The Seventh-day Adventists in Loma Linda, California (USA): Seventh-day Adventists are a very religious group of people. They are strict vegetarians and live in communities tightly knit.

Many studies found that these areas contain extremely high rates of nonagenarians and centenarians, respectively, who are people who exist over 90 and 100 years. Interestingly, genetics probably only accounts for the longevity of 20–30 percent. Environmental influences, including diet and lifestyle, therefore play a huge part in determining your lifespan.

Below are some of the factors of diet and lifestyle which are common to people living in Blue Zones. Blue Zones are districts of the world where people live outstandingly long lives. Studies have found genetics can play a survival function of 20–30 percent.

People Who Exist in Blue Zones Eat a Diet Full of Whole Plant Foods

One thing common to Blue Zones is that those living there eat a plant-based diet of 95 percent primarily. While most of the groups are not strict vegetarians, they tend to eat meat only about five times a month. Several studies have shown that avoiding meat can significantly reduce the risk of death from heart disease, cancer, and several other different causes, including one in more than half a million people.

Alternatively, foods are usually abundant in the following in the Blue Zones:

Vegetables: they are a perfect source of fiber, and many various vitamins and minerals. Eating more than five portions of fruits and vegetables will reduce the risk of heart disease, cancer, and death dramatically a day.

Legumes: Legumes include peas, beans, lentils, and chickpeas, all of which are rich in protein and fiber. Several studies have shown the association between eating legumes and lower mortality.

Whole grains: Whole grains are fiber-rich too. High intakes of whole grains can lower blood pressure and are associated with reduced colorectal cancer and heart disease death.

Nuts: Nuts are great fiber, protein, and polyunsaturated, monounsaturated fat sources. They are associated with reduced mortality in combination with a healthy diet and can even help reverse metabolic syndrome. Some other dietary factors define each Blue Zone.

Some other diet factors that defines each of the blue zones

for example. It is a good origin of omega-3 fats, which is important for the health of the heart and brain. Eating fish in old age is associated with a slower brain decline and reduced heart disease. Citizens in Blue Zones typically eat a plant-based diet of 95 percent that is high in legumes, whole grains, fruits, and nuts, all of which can help to reduce death risk.

The fast and follow the Rule of 80 percent.

Another common habit of the Blue Zones is reduced calorie intake and fasting.

Calories restriction.

Long-term limits on calories can help with longevity. A massive, 25-year study of monkeys found that eating 30 percent less than average calories resulted in significantly longer life. Eating fewer calories in some of the Blue Zones will lead to longer lives. Research in the Okinawans, for example, shows that they were in a calorie deficit before the 1960s, suggesting they were consuming fewer calories than they needed, which may contribute to their longevity.

Okinawans tend to follow the 80 percent law they call "Hara Hachibu," which means they stop consuming when they feel 80 percent full instead of 100 percent full. It stops them from eating too many calories, leading to weight gain and chronic illness. Some studies have also shown that eating slowly, compared to eating quickly, can decrease appetite and improve feelings of fullness. This can be because only 20 minutes after you feed the hormones that make you feel full exceed their highest blood levels.

Therefore, you can eat fewer calories and feel full longer by eating slowly and only until you feel 80 percent full.

Fastsing

While steadily lowering overall calorie intake, intermittent fasting appears helpful to well-being. Icarians, for example, are traditionally Greek Orthodox Christians, a religious group that has many times of the year-round fasting during religious holidays.

One study showed that fasting led to lower blood cholesterol and lower body mass index (BMI) during those religious holidays. It has also been found that many other forms of fasting reduce weight, blood pressure, cholesterol, and many other chronic disease risk factors in humans. These include intermittent fasting, involving day-time fasting or certain days of the week, and fasting-mimicking, involving fasting for a few consecutive days a month.

In Blue Zones, caloric restrictions and periodic fastings are common. Both of these practices can significantly reduce disease risk factors and prolong healthy living conditions.

They drink alcohol in moderation.

Moderate alcohol consumption is another important dietary factor in many of the Blue Zones. There is mixed evidence on whether moderate consumption of alcohol reduces the risk of death. Many studies have shown that taking one to two alcoholic beverages a day can substantially reduce mortality, especially from heart disease.

However, a very recent study suggested that once you take into account other factors in the lifestyle, there is no real effect. The beneficial effect of moderate consumption of alcohol can depend on the type of alcohol. Red wine can be the best type of alcohol since it contains some grape-based antioxidants. In the Icarian and Sardinian Blue Zones, the consumption of one to two glasses of red wine per day is particularly common.

It has been shown that the Sardinian Cannonau wine, made from Grenache grapes, has extremely high levels of antioxidants compared to other wines. Antioxidants help prevent DNA degradation, which can lead to aging. Antioxidants can, therefore, be essential to longevity. A few studies have shown that the association between moderate drinking amounts of red wine and slightly longer life.

As with other research on alcohol consumption, however, it is unclear whether this effect is because wine drinkers appear to have healthier lifestyles too.

Many analyses have shown that people who consumed a 5-ounce (150-ml) glass of wine every day for six months to two years had

31

slightly lower blood pressure, lower blood sugar, higher "healthy" cholesterol, and improved sleep efficiency. It is valuable to note that these effects are considered only for moderate alcohol consumption. Each of these studies also indicated that higher consumption levels increase the risk of death.

In some Blue Zones, people drink one to two glasses of red wine a day, which can help prevent heart disease and reduce death risk.

Exercise is Built Into Daily Life.

Exercise, apart from diet, is another extremely important factor in aging.

People in the Blue Zones do not purposefully exercise by going to the gym. Rather, it is built into their daily lives through gardening, walking, cooking, and other day-to-day tasks. A Sardinian Blue Zone men's study found that their longer life was associated with raising farm animals, living on steeper mountain slopes, and walking long distances to work.

Previously a study of more than 13,000 men showed the benefits of these frequent activities. The amount of distance they were walking or the stories of stairs they were ascending each day measured how long they would survive.

Other studies have demonstrated the benefits of exercise in reducing cancer risk, heart disease, and overall death. The current Physical Activity Guidelines recommendations for Americans suggest a minimum of 75 vigorous-intensity minutes or 150 moderate-intensity minutes of aerobic workout per week. A large analysis, including more than 600,000 people, found that those who were doing the recommended amount of exercise had a 20 percent lower risk of death than those who were not doing physical activity.

Further exercise can reduce the risk of death by as much as 39 percent. Another large study showed that vigorous activity resulted in lower mortality risk than moderate activity. Moderate physical exercise built into everyday life, such as walking and climbing stairs, may help to extend life.

They Get Enough Sleep

Including exercise, it also seems that getting adequate rest and a good night's sleep is very necessary for appreciating a long and healthy life. People in the Blue Zones get enough sleep and often take the naps during the day.

Several analysis has found that not getting enough sleep or having too much sleep will increase the risk of death dramatically, including from heart disease or stroke. A large analysis of 35 studies revealed the optimal sleep duration was seven hours. Sleeping much less or much more than that was linked to an increased risk of death.

People in the Blue Zones tend not to go to sleep, to wake up, or to go to work at set hours. They just sleep the way their body tells them.

Day-time napping is also common in certain Blue Zones, such as Icaria and Sardinia.

Some studies have shown that daytime naps, known as "siestas" in many Mediterranean countries, do not adversely affect the risk of heart disease and death, and may even decrease these risks.

Yet the nap's duration seems to be very significant. Naps of 30 minutes or fewer may be beneficial, but there is an increased risk of heart disease and death associated with anything longer than 30 minutes. People get enough sleep in Blue Zones. Seven hours of night sleep and no more than 30-minute naps during the day can help to reduce the risk of heart disease and death.

Other traits and habits associated with longevity.

Apart from diet, exercise, and rest, the Blue Zones are common to some other social and lifestyle factors, and they can contribute to the longevity of the people living there.

These include:

Being religious or spiritual: usually religious communities are the Blue Zones. Some studies have shown the correlation of being Christian with a lower risk of death. That may be due to social support and lower depression rates.

Having a purpose in life: Blue Zones people tend to have a purpose in life, known as "plan de Vida" or "ikigai" in Okinawa in Nicoya.

This is linked to a lower risk of death, possibly through psychological well-being.

Older and younger alike: Grandparents often live with their families in many Blue Zones. Studies have shown that there is a lower risk of death for grandparents who care for their grandchildren.

A healthy social network: Your social network, in Okinawa called "moai," may affect your health. If your friends are obese, for example, you have a greater risk of becoming obese, possibly through social acceptance of weight gain.

In terms of longevity, factors other than diet and exercise play an important role. Religion, the purpose of life, family, and social networks can also influence how long you're living.

The regions in the Blue Zone are home to some of the world's oldest and healthiest people. Although their lifestyles distinct slightly, they mostly eat a plant-based diet, do regular exercise, drink fair amounts of alcohol, get enough sleep, and have good family, spiritual, and social networking. It has been shown that each of these lifestyle factors is associated with longer life. By embedding them into your lifestyle, you may be able to add a few years to your life.

Over a decade, I've been studying the areas of the world where people live longer and healthier than anywhere else on the planet. Those "Blue Zone" areas are unbelievable because the people living there live longer, even healthier. In inclusion to having a large percentage

35

of people living up to 100, the aging population was also remaining part active well into their 80s and 90s. It typically does not suffer from the degenerative diseases common in most of the industrialized world. I have spent over a decade examining the world's areas where people live longer and healthier lives than anywhere else in the world. Those areas of the "Blue Area" are amazing because the people living there live longer but also healthier.

In addition to having a bigger percentage of people living up to 100, aging people also remain active well into their 90s and 100s. It typically does not suffer from the degenerative diseases common in most industrialized countries. Over a decade, I've been studying the areas of the world where people live longer and healthier than anywhere else on the planet. Those areas of the "Blue Area" are amazing because the people living there live longer but also healthier. While seeing a large percentage of people living up to 100, the aging population remains active well into their 80s and 90s. It is not usually affected by the degenerative diseases prevalent in most industrialized countries. Top Form.

Those areas of the "Green Zone" are amazing because the people living there live longer but also healthier. While seeing a large percentage of people living up to 100, the aging population remains active well into their 80s and 90s. It is not usually affected by the degenerative diseases prevalent in most industrialized countries.

Several individuals, teams, and a team of medical researchers, anthropologists, demographers, and epidemiologists from Blue Zones found common traits of all the Blue Zones regions based on evidence. We call it Power 9:

1. Move naturally. Going spontaneously throughout the day cycling, gardening, doing housework is a central part of living in the Blue Zones.

2. Purpose. It is called ikigai by the Okinawans and is considered scheme de Vida by the Nicoyans. Understanding that you wake up in the morning makes you safer, happier, and adds up to life anticipation of up to seven years.

3. Down shift. Stress is a part of life, but centenarians in the Blue Zones have stress-relieving rituals incorporated into their daily routines. Adventists are praying, Ikarians are naping, and Sardinians are doing a happy hour.

4. 80% rule. People in areas of the Blue Zones stop eating until their stomachs are eighty percent full and consume their smallest meal early in the evening.

5. Plant Slant. Beans are the staple of most centuries-old diets. The rest of the food and meat is served in small amounts of vegetables, fruit, and whole grains.

6. Wein @ 5. Moderate but regular wine intake (with friends and/or food) is part of the lifestyle in the Blue Zones.

7. Belong. Just belong. Being a part of a faith-based community adds to life expectancy four to 14 years.

8. Loved ones first. It is common for centenarians of the Blue Zones to have close and strong family connections (with spouses, parents, grandparents, and grandchildren).

9. Right Tribe. Longest-lived people in the world have close friends and strong social networks.

So if you want to live to be 100, you should dream about omega-3s, kale, and blueberries, there you can eat your way.

People living in the Blue Zones five regions in Europe, Latin America, Asia, and the U.S. researchers have identified themselves as having the highest concentrations of centenarians in the world are moving their bodies a lot. We have social circles that reinforce healthy behaviors. They need some time to de-stress. They're part of most ethnic groups. And they are engaged toward their families.

Chapter 3

Sirtuins And Muscle. Sirtuins And Fat. Sirtuins And Disease

Sirtuins and muscle

Sirtuins have a physiological duty in regulating gene expression and muscle differentiation by detecting changes in the ratio[NADÿ]/[NADH]. SIRT1 suppresses differentiation of myoblasts by deacetylating and inhibiting the MyoD transcription factor. In skeletal muscles, SIRT1 organizes metabolic changes through the deacetylation of PGC-1a required for the activation of genes for the oxidation of mitochondrial fatty acids.

SIRT1 inhibits androgen and regulates androgen receptor function through deacetylation and transcription, thereby influencing muscle mass. It also acts as an important repressor of uncoupling protein-3 (UCP-3), which plays a role in protecting muscle cells against fatty acid overload, reducing the mitochondrial membrane potential, and reducing excessive reactive oxygen species production. In both fetal and adult skeletal muscles, SIRT2 regulates the cell cycle during cell differentiation. It also influences the dynamics of the microtubules by affecting the potential for redox.

Sirtuins and fats.

Sirtuins control a wide variety of processes, including transcription, digestion, and accumulation of fat, neurodegeneration, and aging. The various functions of these proteins were largely ascribed to their ability to catalyze the removal of acetyl groups from other proteins ' lysine amino-acid residues through their deacetylase activity. Yet the sirtuin's exact biological action remains unclear. For example, one sirtuin, SIRT6 that has been involved in stabilizing the genome, inflammation, cancer-cell metabolism, and even lifespan is a very weak deacetylase. Surprisingly, the finding reveals that SIRT6 robustly extracts from lysine residues a myristoyl group— a long-chain fatty-acyl group— and that this biochemical action helps the enzyme to control the secretion of TNF-α, a cytokine protein produced from cells throughout inflammation.

Fatty acids are taken up by transporters of fatty acids by the cell and then transported to mitochondria, where their oxidation contributes to ATP production. To generate ketone bodies, HMGCS2 breaks down the fatty acids. In the cytosol, lipogenesis (dashed arrows) assists in the synthesis of malonyl CoA fatty acids by fatty acid synthase, after which they are processed into triglycerides. When the energy demand is high, lipolysis will break down triglycerides to release fatty acids, mostly in fat tissue. Instead, these are absorbed into the bloodstream. SIRT1 reduces fatty acid storage by enhancing lipolysis through

41

PPAR-g inhibition and by decreasing fatty acid synthesis through SREBP1c. SIRT6 represses gene expression involved in the synthesis of fatty acids. SIRT3 activates LCAD to boost oxidation at b. SIRT3 promotes the production of ketones in the body by activating HMGCS2. SIRT3 stimulates the reduction of ROS in SOD2. SIRT3 enhances cellular respiration by increasing the I, Complex II, Complex III, and IDH2 activities. SIRT4 appears to be a negative transcription regulator of genes involved in the oxidation of fatty acids.

Lipid metabolism.

SIRT1 regulates a series of lipid-metabolism related proteins and genes. A metabolic shift from lipid combination and storage to lipolysis is observed under the condition of fasting or short-term food deprivation, the features of which include decreased levels of ATP and NADH. With further research, under the fasting condition, SIRT1 was found to repress lipid synthesis and promote lipolysis in response to this typical alteration. The detailed mechanism related to how SIRT1 exerts its impact on lipid metabolism in these two processes is discussed separately in the following sense.

Lipids synthesis.

SIRT1 is shown to play a role in the down-regulation of both SREBP-1 and SREBP-2 during fasting, which results in lipid synthesis inhibition and fat storage. Until activation, SREBPs remain attached to the nuclear envelope and endoplasmic reticulum membranes. SREBPs undergo cleavage-induced activation and translocation to the nucleus when cellular sterol levels are low, and promote the transcription of enzymes that are important for sterol biosynthesis. Additionally, resveratrol activation of SIRT1 correlates with the increase of AMP-activated protein kinase (AMPK), a nutrient-sensing molecule that inhibits the synthesis of fatty acid.

Lipolysis

In white adipose tissue, SIRT1 obligate to and keep back PPARπ activity by docking co-repressors, nuclear receptor co-repressor (NCoR), and retinoid and thyroid hormone receptor (SMRT) silencing mediator. The SIRT1/PPARπ/NCoR complex is recruited in the promoter region of target genes for specific DNA sequences and inhibits their transcription. This effect can have negative effects on genes involved in the accumulation of fatty acids and the promotion of lipolysis. By favoring energy movement from white adipose tissue and oxidation in tissues such as brown adipose tissue, SIRT1 can alter the status of cellular energy production. Additionally, SIRT1 may be

43

induced to activate fatty acid oxidation genes in fasting liver, and PGC-1α deacetylates, which promote the use of fatty acids.

Cholesterol transport.

SIRT1 encourages survival in organisms ranging from yeast to mammals, and these defensive acts are thought to derive, at least in part, from beneficial energy control and metabolic homeostasis. High cholesterol levels have a significant impact on mortality, and a recent study indicates a correlation between cholesterol and SIRT1, which gives further indication of the lifetime prolongation role of SIRT1. SIRT1−/− mice showed significant decreases in total plasma cholesterol levels, HDL cholesterol levels, and triglyceride levels, indicating that SIRT1 is a positive liver X receptor regulator (LXR). SIRT1 deacetylates LXR on lysine 432 and then promotes its ubiquitination, resulting in the efflux of cell cholesterol. LXR activation is beneficial in that it not only inhibits the absorption of intestinal cholesterol and promotes the transport of reverse cholesterol but also exerts potent anti-inflammatory effects that involve trans-repression. Until now, it remains doubtful to what extent the LXR deacetylation mediated by SIRT1 can affect these anti-inflammatory effects.

Growing evidence suggests thatSIRT1is a key regulator for the metabolism of glucose and lipids. Through its deacetylase activity, it can regulate glucose and lipid metabolism by deacetylating certain

44

proteins. SIRT1may be a new therapeutic target for the prevention of glucose-and lipid metabolism-related diseases.

Sirtuins and diseases

Abbreviations

Aβ Amyloid-β;

AADPR acetyl-ADP ribose;

AASIS amino acid-stimulated insulin secretion;

AceCS2 acetyl coenzyme A synthetase 2;

AD Alzheimer's disease;

AR androgen receptor;

BAT brown adipose tissue;

BER base excision repair;

CoA coenzyme A;

CR caloric restriction;

FOXO forkhead box type O transcription factor;

GDH glutamate dehydrogenase;

HD Huntington's disease;

HDAC histone deacetylase;

MEF mouse embryonic fibroblast;

NAD nicotinamide adenine dinucleotide;

NADH reduced nicotinamide adenine dinucleotide;

NFκB nuclear factor κB;

Nmnat 1 nicotinamide mononucleotide adenyltransferase 1;

PGC-1α peroxisome proliferator-activated receptor γ coactivator 1α;

PolyQ polyglutamine;

PPARγ peroxisome proliferator-activated receptor γ;

Sir2p silent information regulator two protein;

UCP uncoupling protein.

Sirtuins regulate multiple vital functions and are involved in some pathologies, including metabolic diseases, neurodegenerative disorders, and cancer. SirT1 has been demonstrated to be significantly up-regulated in various cancer types, including acute myeloid leukemia (AML), prostate, colon, and skin cancer.

THE RISING OCCURENCE of obesity-related diseases, such as dyslipidemia, diabetes, and cardiovascular and cerebrovascular diseases, has become a bigger public health issue in industrialized countries. Many therapeutic and preventive strategies have seen the light of day to prevent or combat obesity, but few have to get through the test of time. Another observation that caught attention in this sense is the so-called "French paradox." First reported in 1819 by Irish mathematician Samuel Black, the French paradox alludes to the fact that the French are viewed as having a relatively low incidence of cardiovascular and metabolic diseases, while their diet is high in saturated fat. One of the primary factors leading to this comparative benefit is believed to be the heavy intake of red wine, which is abundant in polyphenol resveratrol.

In the meantime, it has also been well known since the 1930s that caloric restriction (CR) can slow the aging process and delay the onset of various age-related diseases, such as cancer, cardiovascular diseases, and metabolic diseases. CR extends lifespan significantly in organisms ranging from yeast and nematodes to rodents and monkeys. CR's beneficial health outcomes are remarkably similar to those caused by resveratrol in many animal models, indicating that the molecular mechanisms through which resveratrol operates are identical to those triggered by CR. It has been proposed recently that the sirtuins could be the specific mediators that explain both the effects of CR pathways and resveratrol. In this review, we will talk about the molecular mechanism underlying these sirtuins ' biological activity, their functional roles in the physiology of the whole body, and their possible associations with human diseases.

Adp-Ribosyl Transferases or Nicotinamide Adenine Dinucleotide-Dependent Histone Deacetylases are sirtuins.

The founding part of a group of the sirtuin protein family was Saccharomyces cerevisiae silent information regulator two proteins (Sir2p), a Nicotinamide adenine dinucleotide (NAD+)-dependent histone deacetylase (HDAC) that regulates the silencing of chromatin. Yeast strains with abnormal Sir2p levels exhibit defects in many cellular functions, including silencing transcription and

47

recombination, senescence, and repairing DNA. To S. In addition to Sir2p, there are four sirtuins (NAD+-dependent histone deacetylases Hst1–Hst4), whereas, in mammals, there are seven homologs (i.e., SIRT1–SIRT7, indicated (Table 1). The remarkable preservation of sirtuin gene family members from yeast to humans indicates that these proteins are playing vital physiological roles.

Table 1.

Main Characteristic of Mammalian Sirtuins

The sirtuins were originally classified as Class III HDACs among the large HDAC protein family. While groups I and II HDACs use zinc as a cofactor and are inhibited by trichostatin A, sirtuins are not inhibited by trichostatin A and transform acetylated protein substrates in a reaction using NAD+ into a deacetylated protein, nicotinamide, and 2'-O-and 3'-O-acetyl-ADPR (AADPR) acetyl ester metabolites, which are formed by the transition of the acetyl group to the ADP-ribose port The activity of the sirtuins deacetylase is regulated by the ratio of cell[NAD+]/[NADH], i.e., NAD+ acts as an activator. In contrast, nicotinamide and reduced adenine dinucleotide (NADH) inhibits its activity.

Two Reactions The Sirtuins Catalyzed, i.e., Deacetylation and ADP-Ribosylation Sirtuins (SIRT1–SIRT3, SIRT5) catalyze a deacetylation reaction in which an acetyl group is transmitted to the NAD+ and a 2′-O-acetyl-ADPR moiety of ADP-ribose (ADPR). The 3′-O-acetyl-ADPR is formed from 2′-O-acetyl-ADPR non-enzymatically. Conversely, SIRT4, and SIRT6 catalyze protein ADP-ribosylation instead of deacetylation.

Since sirtuins are class III HDACs, it was logical that their function was initially related to the transcriptional constraint. Acetylated histones H1, H4, and H3, are known as physiological substrates for the sirtuins, and lysine 16 appears to be the most critical residue for sirtuin-mediated transcriptional silencing in histone H4. Afterward, it has been noted that the sirtuins also deacetylate a growing number of nonhistone proteins, extending their biological functions to a large extent. These nonhistone sirtuin substrates involve several transcriptional regulators such as the enzymes, acetyl coenzyme A (CoA) synthetase 2 (AceCS2), but also coactivator 1α (PGC-1α) and structural proteins such as α-tubulin (Table 1), such as the coactivator 1α (PGC-1α), forkhead box type O transcription factors (FOXO), and the peroxisome proliferator-activated receptor ÿ (PPPARπ).

Interestingly, AADPR, a product generated by the sirtuins catalyzed in the deacetylation reaction, also plays a role as a second messenger since it is involved in establishing a transcriptionally silent and

49

functionally heterochromatic state. AADPR achieves this effect through two independent mechanisms involving, on the one hand, a conformational change in SIRT1, which potentiates the gene-silencing effects of the Sir complex in a feedforward loop, and, on the other, the binding to the histone variant macro H2A1.1, present in inactive heterochromatic regions. Because the cellular[NAD+]/[NADH] ratio, nicotinamide, and AADPR levels are controlled by cellular energetics, SIRT1 can be an extremely versatile energy sensor that enables transcription to sense the cell's metabolic state.

Two sirtuins, SIRT4 and SIRT6, lack substantial deacetylase activity but have a strong NAD+-dependent ADP-ribosyl transferase activity instead (Fig. 1). Given the initial report on the enzymatic behavior of yeast Sir2p, which identified a mono-ADP-ribosyl transferase function, the ADP-ribosyl transferase activities of those two SIRTs are not a complete surprise. Posttranslational modification of protein substrates by mono-ADP-ribosylation requires the formation of an N- or S-glycosidic association between a particular amino acid (such as arginine or cysteine) on the acceptor protein and NAD+ ADP-ribose residue.

The seven mammalian sirtuins show significant homology in sequence and contain preserved catalytic and NAD+ binding domains (Fig. 2 and Table 1). Although eukaryotic sirtuins were divided into

50

four broad phylogenetic groups based on sequence similarities, with SIRT1, SIRT2, and SIRT3 composing class I, SIRT4 composing class II, SIRT5 forming class III, and SIRT6 and SIRT7 forming class IV, there is no obvious correlation between this classification and the sirtuin's specific biological functions. Another more relevant way of classifying the sirtuins functionally is based on their intracellular localization (Table 1). Four sirtuins are nuclear proteins, SIRT1, SIRT3, SIRT6, and SIRT7, but their subnuclear localizations are distinct. SIRT1 is detected in the nuclei but excluded from the nuclei, while SIRT6 and SIRT7, respectively, are associated with heterochromatic regions and nucleoli. In general, SIRT2 is located in the cytoplasm but binds chromatin in the nucleus during the G2/M phase. The mitochondria contain SIRT3, SIRT4, and SIRT5. While initially described as a mitochondrial protein, recent studies suggest that SIRT3 may also be a nuclear protein that moves during cell stress to the mitochondria. However, the exact localization of the SIRT3–SIRT5 in the mitochondria has not yet been experimentally defined.

All seven sirtuins are omnipresent in human tissues, although for most sirtuins, higher levels of mRNA expression are discovered in the brain and testis. Except for SIRT5 and SIRT2, the expression for the sirtuins is higher in fetal compared to the adult brain, which may suggest the likelihood that they will play important roles in neuronal system development.

51

Cell Proliferation Control and Sirtuins, Stress Resistance, and Cancer.

Several factors controlling cell proliferation and apoptosis are known as substrates for sirtuin, such as p53. SIRT1 is reported to be associated with protein p53, a tumor suppressor. P53 has several acetylation sites, which stabilizes and triggers its hyperacetylation to cause apoptosis and cell cycle arrest. Conversely, SIRT1's deacetylation of p53 is predicted to induce its destruction through the ubiquitin-mediated MDM2 (mouse double minute 2) pathway. In fact, in response to DNA damage and oxidative stress, overexpression ofSIRT1 inhibits p53 transcriptional activity and p53-dependent apoptosis, whereas overexpression of the dominant-negative SIRT1 protein may potentiate these cellular stress responses. The levels of p53 acetylation were somewhat up-regulated in thymocytes from SIRT1-deficient mice after exposure to ionizing radiation, indicating that SIRT1 plays a role in increasing the stress resistance of the cells. Increased p53 acetylation was associated with senescence, too. Interestingly, SIRT1 has recently been shown to promote replicative senescence through a process involving p19ARF, which by inhibiting MDM2, positively regulates p53. This effect contrasts markedly with the Sir2p function in yeast, which extends the lifespan of replicates.

Sirtuins also affect transcription factor activity in the FOXO family. Genetic epistasis in Caenorhabditis elegans and metabolic research in mice indicate that FOXO genes regulate cell differentiation, transformation, and metabolism. For C. Elegans, FOXO orthology mutation Daf16 (abnormal period formation) rescues the permanent state, caused by insulin / IGF orthology mutations Daf2. In mammalian cells, phosphatidylinositol3-kinase growth-factor-induced activation leads to increased serine/threonine kinase AKT / protein kinase B activity, which in turn leads to phosphorylation and inactivation of FOXO proteins through their retention in the cytoplasm. In response to oxidative stress, the translocation of FOXO3a from the cytoplasm into the nucleus is caused by its deacetylation by SIRT1. SIRT1 and deacetylated FOXO3a form a complex within the nucleus that promotes cell-cycle arrest and tolerance to oxidative stress but inhibits FOXO3a's capacity to induce apoptosis. SIRT1-mediated deacetylation also affects the nucleocytoplasmic shuttling of FOXO1, which results in the expression of target genes of FOXO1, thus inducing gluconeogenesis and hepatocyte release of glucose.

SIRT1 is also reported to play a significant role in differentiating myocytes. Throughout muscle differentiation, the rates of SIRT1 and the[NAD+]/[NADH] ratio decrease. SIRT1 over-expression retards muscle differentiation through the development of an acetyltransferase PCAF (p300/CBP-associated factor) and MyoD complex while muscle gene expression and differentiation are improved in cells with decreased SIRT1 expression. Alternatively,

SIRT1 inactivates the muscle cell transcription factor, the myocyte enhancer factor MEF2 via deacetylation. SIRT1 was also reported to bind and deacetylate the androgen receptor (AR) to a conserved lysine motif, thereby keep back the ligand-induced AR transcriptional activity by inhibiting coactivator-induced interactions between the AR amino and carboxyl termini.

Hst2, the SIRT2 yeast orthology, can induce Sir2p-independent lifespan extension and rDNA silencing in yeast, demonstrating the SIRT's redundancies in yeast lifespan regulation. As for mammalian SIRT2, some substrates, including α-tubulin and histone H4K16Ac, are deacetylated. SIRT2 had been shown to play an important role in controlling the cell cycle in mammalian cell culture systems. In the S and G2 phase, global levels of H4K16 acetylation peak dropping before cells enter mitosis, coinciding with the growth expression of SIRT2, its nuclear translocation, and chromatin association. In embryonic fibroblasts (MEFs) of the mouse with SIRT2 deficiency, H4K16 acetylation remains high during mitosis, delaying entry into S-phase. This indicates that the conversion of H4K16Ac to its deacetylated form, regulated by SIRT2, may be key to the production of condensed chromatin. It was also suggested that SIRT2 act as a gene for tumor suppressors in human gliomas. Gliomas often experience down-regulation of the SIRT2 gene expression and/or deletion of the chromosomal region harboring the SIRT2 gene. Thus,

SIRT2 expression could serve as a potential molecular diagnostic marker for gliomas, and modulation of its activity could be of interest to gliomas management.

The SIRT6 nuclear protein is a weak deacetylase but is endowed with the robust activity of ADP-ribosyltransferase. SIRT6−/− MEFs have an increased frequency of miscellaneous chromosomal aberrations, indicating that SIRT6 contributes to maintaining the integrity of genomes. The deficiency of SIRT6 also impairs the proliferation of these MEFs and increases their sensitivity to DNA-damaging substances. This SIRT6 regulation of genomic stability is linked to its function in the repair of single-stranded DNA breaks by base excision (BER). Interestingly, those defects are rescued by overexpression of the DNA polymerase involved in BER, Polβ. SIRT6−/− Mice die prematurely from several rather acute degenerative processes, containing the loss of sc fat, cutback of bone mineral density, colitis, and lymphopenia combined with increased apoptosis of the lymphocytes. SIRT6 may also control metabolism since SIRT6−/− mice exhibits low serum IGF-I levels and a gradual decline in serum glucose. However, it remains unclear how SIRT6 influences BER, and whether SIRT6−/− mice's altered serum IGF and insulin levels directly contribute to aging phenotypes or reflect compensatory changes.

SIRT7 is a nucleolar protein in which active rRNA genes interact with RNA polymerase I. SIRT7 increases rRNA transcription overexpression, while its down-regulation decreases rRNA transcription overexpression. Surprisingly, the expression of SIRT7 is elevated in tissues that have a high potential for proliferation, such as liver, spleen, and testis. This contrasts with tissues with low cellular turnover, such as the skeletal and heart muscle and brain that express low SIRT7 levels. Thus, SIRT7 appears to drive ribosome biogenesis in cell division, and it has been associated with thyroid and breast cancer. SIRT7 gene explanation is up-regulated in these cancers, and its levels are also closely linked to tumor development and breast cancer disease progression. However, further study will be required to identify the mechanism underlying the enhanced expression of the SIRT7 gene in these cancers.

All of these combined studies suggest significant sirtuin functions in cell proliferation control: SIRT1 inhibits p53 and modulates FOXO function, SIRT2 regulates chromosome condensation throughout the cell cycle, SIRT6 works in BER, while SIRT7 stimulates rRNA transcription.

Sirtuins supervise the metabolic activity.

The fact that various of the protein substrates involved in metabolism, such as AceCS2 and PGC-1α, which are deacetylated by the sirtuins, suggested a metabolic role for this family of proteins. This hypothesis has been substantiated by studies using both cell-based approaches and a combination of entirely animal genetic and pharmacological approaches.

Two groups reported the germline phenotypesSIRT1−/− mice, showing some similarities but also revealing differences, potentially the result of the methods used to generate the mice. SIRT1−/− mice were generally smaller at birth and displayed a high postnatal lethality due to developmental problems not found in yeast, C. Elegant, Drosophila, or. Some of the SIRT1−/− mice lived to maturity in an outbred context, but they have fertility problems and show some other disorders, including skeletal, leg, and heart defects. Studying some of these genetically engineered SIRT1 mouse models revealed a role for SIRT1 in the homeostasis of the pancreatic. SIRT1 was preferentially clustered in the Langerhans islets in the pancreas. In SIRT1−/− mice, glucose reaction insulin secretion was smaller than wild-type littermates, suggesting that SIRT1 positively controls insulin secretion in pancreatic β-cells.

Conversely, β-cell-specific SIRT1-overexpressing transgenic mice display improved glucose tolerance and decreased insulin secretion induced by glucose. From the microarray study contrasting patterns of gene expression in pancreatic β-cell lines SIRT1-overexpressing-and knockdown, uncoupling protein (UCP2), a protein that negatively

57

regulates insulin discharge in pancreatic β-cells, was identified as a target that has been repressed by SIRT 1. SIRT1 reduces UCP2 gene expression by binding directly to the promoter UCP2, resulting in a greater pairing of mitochondrial respiration and ATP synthesis that will trigger insulin secretion.

PPARÿ is a crucial regulator for adipogenesis and accumulation of fat by regulating the expression of many adipocyte-specific genes. SIRT1 effectively represses PPARÿ by docking with two of its corepressors, NcoR (nuclear corepressor) and SMRT (Retinoid and thyroid hormone receptor silencing mediator). Therefore, it was suggested that SIRT1 act as a corepressor of the transcription mediated by PPARI'. From a practical point of view, SIRT1's PPARÿ inhibition attenuates adipogenesis, and SIRT1's up-regulation causes lipolysis and fat loss in differentiated fat cells. Conversely, reducing the expression of SIRT1 in SIRT1+/− mice thus jeopardizes the mobilization of adipose tissue fatty acids during fasting.

The cofactor PGC-1α, the main regulator of mitochondrial biogenesis, is perhaps the most relevant target for SIRT1 in the metabolic arena. Deacetylation mediated by the SIRT1 activates PGC-1α. Activating PGC-1α in the liver will facilitate the gluconeogenic activity of hepatocyte nuclear factor 4α and stimulate the output of hepatic glucose. The SIRT1-mediated deacetylation of PGC-1α is converted into improved mitochondrial production in the muscle and brown

58

adipose tissue (BAT), which has resulted in increased stress resistance and thermogenesis, resulting in defense against the development of obesity and connected metabolic dysfunctions. SIRT1 strictly depends on cellular NAD+ levels for its deacetylase activity, which reflects cellular energy status. The changes in the cellular NAD+ levels affecting the activity of SIRT1 deacetylase thus seem to inform PGC-1α about the status of cellular energy. Then PGC-1α can adapt the production of cellular energy through its commanding role in the biogenesis and function of mitochondrial. Such studies position SIRT1, which acts as a sensor of cellular energy, as an essential regulator of mitochondrial function upstream of PGC-1α.

It is clear that many of these researches, which focused on a given type of tissue, indicated potential linkages between metabolic homeostasis and action on SIRT1. As mentioned, SIRT1 stimulates insulin secretion by repressing UCP2 in response to glucose in the pancreas; in the liver, SIRT1 promotes gluconeogenesis and suppresses glycolysis; in adipose tissue, SIRT1 prevents fat storage and improves lipolysis by repressing PPARπ. These pleiotropic, frequently opposing, metabolic effects of SIRT1 in different tissues complicated the elucidation of SIRT1's impact on metabolic homeostasis in the whole body. Two recent studies using the resveratrol SIRT1 activator have shed more light on this complex function of SIRT1 in metabolism. Resveratrol has been shown in one study to model some features of CR in mice on a high-calorie diet by prolonging the lifetime, enhancing insulin sensitivity, and increasing motor function. This research thus expands previous work that resveratrol mimics CR activation of SIRT1 and slows aging in a wide range of species that derive from S. Cerevisiae > C. Drosophila elegant. Treatment of mice with a bigger dose of resveratrol was also shown in a second independent study to shield them from diet-induced obesity and the resulting insulin resistance. This study showed that SIRT1-mediated PGC-1α deacetylation linked the amelioration of insulin sensitivity to an enhanced mitochondrial function following activation of PGC-1α. Also, enhanced mitochondrial activity has led to an increase in oxidative muscle type fibers and increased muscle fatigue resistance. Furthermore, a significant association between three single-nucleotide polymorphisms in the SIRT1 gene and energy homeostasis in humans indicated that SIRT1 is an attractive and validated target for regulating energy and metabolic homeostasis in humans. SIRT3 was genuinely thought to be a mitochondrial protein, but it has recently been shown to be a mitochondrial transfer from its normal nuclear homeostasis SIRT3 expression is finely regulated. In mice, SIRT3 expression levels in white adipose tissue and BAT are up-regulated by caloric restriction (CR). Cold weather triggers SIRT3 in BAT too. Interestingly, SIRT3's constitutive expression promotes the expression of PGC-1α, UCP1, and other genes involved in mitochondrial works, indicating that SIRT3 modulates adaptive thermogenesis in BAT, a process which most likely involves both nuclear and mitochondrial activities. One SIRT3 mitochondrial activity is the deacetylation and activation of the mitochondrial form of AceCS2, an enzyme that catalyzes the formation of acetate CoA. The deacetylation of AceCS2 thus increases the conversion of acetate into acetyl CoA, a cycle of tricarboxylic acid intermediates. AceCS2 is abundantly found in the heart and skeletal muscle but is absent from the liver, and its expression is triggered when the energy is reduced, as during CR and ketogenesis. Since SIRT3 promotes the metabolic use of acetate, maintaining energy production under conditions where ATP is scarce can thus be particularly important. SIRT1 deacetylates and stimulates the cytoplasmic AceCS1 in analogy to this role of SIRT3 to provide acetyl CoA, which serves as a building block for fatty acid and synthesis of cholesterols. For one of the human sirtuins only, i.e., SIRT3, a direct genetic link was identified to longevity. Mutations were enriched in long-lived individuals in the SIRT3 gene enhancer, which up-regulates its expression.

Another SIRT-protein, SIRT4, was recently shown to interact with glutamate dehydrogenase (GDH). In the mitochondria, glutamate formed from glutamine is converted by GDH to the intermediate cycle of tricarboxylic acid α-ketoglutarate. It facilitates mitochondrial activity and raises the ATP / ADP ratio, which then stimulates insulin secretion of β-cells in the pancreatic. Uses NAD+ for ADP-ribosylate and decreases GDH activity, thus reducing α-ketoglutarate production and ATP generation. GDH activity increases in SIRT4-deficient pancreatic β-cells, leading to a stimulation of insulin secretion in response to glutamine. Therefore SIRT4 has an inhibitory effect on the insulin secretion triggered by amino acids (AASIS). Speculating that AASIS is activated during chronic CR seems reasonable because protein turnover is raised, and amino acids are used as energy and carbon sources to urge gluconeogenesis in this condition. By this, GDH repressionSIRT4 is alleviated during long-term CR, resulting in activation of AASIS in β-cells and potentially in liver gluconeogenesis. CR thus reducesSIRT4 activity, which is contrary to SIRT1 activity being triggered during CR. Also, SIRT4 and SIRT1 exert negative and positive control over insulin secretion, respectively, which is striking given that both of their activities are controlled by one metabolite, i.e., AND+.

Axonal degeneration is an important morphological feature found in both peripheral neuropathies and neurodegenerative diseases, such as Alzheimer's disease (AD) and amyotrophic lateral sclerosis. In degenerative processes, axonal degeneration usually occurs at the early stage and often precedes or closely correlates with clinical symptoms such as cognitive decay.

There are several reports in the neuronal system which support an axonal protective role for SIRT1. At the distal ration of a transected axon, which is called Wallerian degeneration, a self-destructive degeneration process is observed Wallerian slow degeneration (wlds) is a line of the mouse with delayed axonal degeneration in response to the axonal lesion. This phenomenon is thought to be gotten from the overexpression of a chimerical nuclear molecule (Wlds protein) corresponding to the full-length nicotinamide mononucleotide adenyltransferase 1 (Nmnat 1), an enzyme required for both NAD+ biosynthesis de novo and salvage pathways (Fig. 3), and a short region of a ubiquitin fusion degradation protein 2a. In a recent study, Nmnat 1 overexpression alone could prevent axonal degeneration, indicating that Nmnat 1's protective effect could be mediated by an increase in NAD+ neuronal reserve and/or SIRT1 activity.

NAD+ Biosynthesis Super Pathway in Mammals NAD+ is synthesized through two major pathways, the de salvage and Novo pathways, and these two pathways converge at mononucleotide nicotinic acid. The moiety of NAD+ nicotinic acid is synthesized from tryptophan via the kynurenine pathway on the de novo pathway. NAD+ is generated by recycling its degradation product such as nicotinamide in the NAD + salvage pathway. ART, ADP-ribosyl transferase; nicotinic acid, NA; NAAD, nicotinic adenine dinucleotide; NAM, nicotinic acid mononucleotide; NaMN, nicotinic

63

acid mononucleotide; Nampt, nicotinamide phosphoribosyltransferase; NMN, nicotinic acid mononucleotide; NPT, nicotinic acid phosphoribosyltransferase; NR, nicotinamide riboside; Nrk, nicotinamide riboside kinase; PARP, poly-ADP-polymeraseaseesis; PBEF,

It is well known that in mouse models of AD and Parkinson's disease, CR protects neurons from degeneration, and SIRT1 might facilitate neuronal survival. While caloric intake and insulin sensitivity are documented to be associated with AD, the mechanism underlying those relations is not yet completely understood (98, 99). AD's diagnosis is characterized by the presence of amyloid plaques, neurofibrillary intracellular tangles, and marked cell death. The amyloid plaque consists of amyloid-β (Aβ) peptide, which is sequentially cleaved by β-secretase and ÿ-secretase (101–103) from the amyloid precursor protein. This abnormal deposition of Aβ peptide inside the brain is the hallmark of AD neuropathology, and accumulation of aggregated Aβ is hypothesized to initiate a pathological cascade resulting in the onset and progression of AD. Aβ peptides can induce microglia NFÿB activity via TNF-receptor type 1 or advanced glycation end-product receptor. The activation of SIRT1 or the administration of the SIRT1 activator resveratrol significantly decreases the signaling of this NFÿB. This strongly implies that SIRT1 can attenuate Aβ-stimulated neurotoxicity and inflammatory

64

responses related to AD by inhibiting microglial NFπB signals. Also, SIRT1 is intended to prevent the generation of Aβ peptide by promoting the nonamyloidogenic processing of amyloid precursor protein by inhibiting the expression of Rho-kinase 1.

In addition to this inflammatory something falling leading to neuronal cell death, another intrinsic pathway of cell death, i.e., the cell death pathway based on mitochondria, is attracting attention in the context of AD. Besides, Aβ peptides, which can directly reach the inner membrane of the mitochondria, can bind to a protein called Aβ-binding alcohol dehydrogenase called a mitochondrial-matrix and guide to the mitochondria. It reduces the production of ATP and decreases the production of oxygen radicals, which may ultimately trigger mitochondrial-dependent cell death as weakened mitochondria are unable to sustain the cells ' energy demands. Consistent with these findings, a close interaction between Aβ and the inner mitochondrial membrane has been documented in AD mouse models along with increased free-radical generation and decreased cytochrome c oxidase activity. In AD, SIRT1 could contribute to this process through its stimulating activity on mitochondria.

The mitochondrial insufficiency is also observed in Huntington's disease (HD), another neurodegenerative disease. HD patients are characterized by marked decreases in glucose metabolism and increased lactate levels in the basal ganglia, reduced activity of several

65

key components of oxidative phosphorylation pathways in the striatal neuron mitochondria, and pronounced morphological abnormalities, including disorder of the mitochondrial matrix and cristae. The mutant huntingtin protein is expected to link these mitochondrial dysfunctions with dysregulation of PGC-1α transcription and/or activity. Because recent reports show that SIRT1 regulates PGC-1α activity and because some of the sirtuins control some aspects of mitochondrial metabolism, sirtuin activity modulation could be an interesting approach for the therapy of these neurodegenerative diseases. Besides, the ability of such a strategy has been validated in HD models for nematode and neuronal cell lines for the mouse. In these models, the extended polyglutamine (PolyQ) pathway was shown to cause PolyQ-dependent neuronal dysfunction in HD-associated huntingtin (htt) protein. This abnormality caused by the PolyQ mutant could be rescued by SIRT1 overexpression or by treatment with resveratrol. Sirtuin inhibitors, such as nicotinamide or sirtinol, suppressed this favorable effect, directly proving that SIRT1 activation could be useful in HD.

Perspectives.

In several model organisms varying from yeast to mouse, the founding member of the sirtuin family, Sir2p in yeast or Sir2p in mammals, has now been well conclusively proved as a key molecule that influence longevity within the context of CR. However, the mechanisms involved may be distinct in the various species. The vital function that the sirtuins play in the control of the cellular metabolism indicated that they could be important determinants of the metabolism of the whole body and protect against many chronic diseases associated with metabolism. Likewise, potential sirtuin applications in neuronal cell survival and response to stress and cell cycle control indicate the potential importance of this gene family in neurodegenerative disease and cancer pathogenesis. Additional insight into the sirtuin's biological actions will require an in vivo definition of the exact roles of each gene family member with appropriate genetic, pharmacological, and physiological instruments. Once this is achieved, a select member of the sirtuins is expected to become interesting potential targets for future therapies against age-related illness.

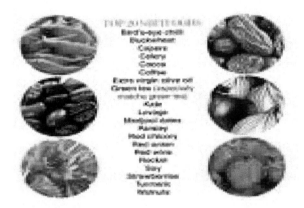

What is the Sirtfood diet?

As the latest crazy diet, a diet rich in' sirt foods,' everybody is talking about it. These special foods work by activating specific proteins known as sirtuins in the body. Sirtuins are thought to prevent the body's cells from dying when under stress, and are thought to control inflammation, metabolism, and aging processes. Sirtuins affect the capacity of the body to burn fat and improve the metabolism, resulting in a weight loss of seven pounds per week while retaining muscle.

Sirtfoods are plant foods which are rich in specific polyphenols which activate our sirtuin genes. Eating these sirt foods turns on a process of recycling in our cells to clear up all the clutter and waste that grows up with age and normally causes ill health. Our cells tap into our fat stores to fuel that recycling process. It resulted in rejuvenated cells, a lack of fitness, strength and weight.

-Sirtuins are master of metabolic regulators that control our ability to burn fat and stay healthy

-Sirtuins act as energy sensors within our cells and are activated when a shortage of energy is detected

-Both Fasting and exercise activate our sirtuin genes but can be hard to persevere with and may have drawbacks

The Top 20 Sirtfoods

Buckwheat

Capers

Celery

Chilli

Chocolate

Coffee

Extra Virgin Olive Oil

Green Tea – ideally matcha

Kale

Lovage

Medjool Dates

Parsley

Red Chicory

Red Onion

Red Wine

Rocket

Soy

Strawberries

Turmeric

Walnuts

The Sirtfood diet introduces a completely new group of Superfoods. They have the name Sirtfoods, because they contain substances that activate Sirtuin or 'skinny' genes, the same genes as exercise and fasting.

Sirtfoods are the innovative way our sirtuin genes can be regulated in the best way possible. These are the particularly rich wonder foods in unique natural plant chemicals, called polyphenols, which have the ability to activate our sirtuin genes by clicking on them. Essentially, they emulate the results of fasting and exercise and thus offer impressive benefits by helping the body better regulate blood sugar levels, burning fat, building muscle, and improving wellbeing and memory.

Because they are stationary, plants have developed a highly sophisticated system of stress-response and produced polyphenols to help them adapt to their environment's challenges. When we eat these plants, we also eat these nutrients of polyphenol. They have a profound effect: they activate our own innate pathways of stress-response.

While all plants have stress-response systems, only some have evolved to produce remarkable amounts of polyphenols which activate sirtuin. These are sirt-foods. Their finding means that there is now a revolutionary new way to trigger the sirtuin genes, instead of rigid fasting regimens or arduous exercise programs: consuming an ample diet of sirt foods. Most of all, the diet involves putting food (sirt) on your plate, and not getting it off.

Let's check out their health benefits

1. Buckwheat

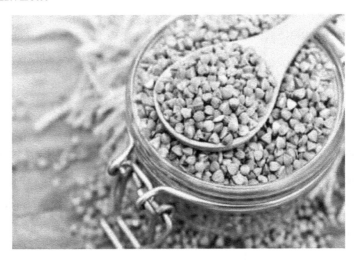

While the name may suggest otherwise, buckwheat is not in fact a form of wheat. And it's not a plant at all. This plant is widely grown in Asia and can be used for a variety of culinary purposes, particularly in noodles, breakfast foods and some drinks. This is also used for those eating a raw diet in recettes. In fact, Buckwheat is a seed derived from the plant Fagopyrum esculentum, which remains short but becomes very widespread and develops green heart-shaped leaves with tiny white flowers. Cultivated in Asia and parts of Europe and North America as a grain-like seed and cover crop, the plant's seeds are commonly referred to as pseudocereals. The seeds are rich in protein and fiber, as well as a variety of antioxidants and other nutrients, leading many to consider buckwheat as a superfood.

What Are The Nutritional Benefits Of Buckwheat?

1. Improved Heart Health

The Grain-like seed helps to decrease inflammation and lower levels of LDL, or "bad cholesterol," both of which are important to maintain heart health. Rutin, a form of phytonutrient and antioxidant that helps stabilize blood pressure and suppress cholesterol, is the main nutrient that offers such cardiovascular benefits.

2. Reduced Blood Sugar

The pseudocereal is very small on the glycemic index—the means that the carbohydrate content is gradually ingested into the bloodstream, creating a constant flow of energy for your body. This healthy seed helps with diabetes management by avoiding a sudden spike in blood sugar, and may boost insulin resistance.

3. Gluten Free And Non-Allergenic

While it can be used as whole grains such as wheat and barley, this seed is inherently gluten-free, making it a great alternative for people with celiac disease or allergy to food. Swapping this seed with traditional gluten-containing grains can also be helpful for people with intestinal problems, such as leaky gut syndrome.

73

4. Rich In Dietary Fiber

This food provides 6 grams of dietary fibre for each cup serving of cooked groats. Dietary fiber helps keep food moving smoothly through the digestive tract, and can help you feel fuller longer–this can be an advantage if you try to lose weight.

5. Protects Against Cancer

This pseudocereal contains antioxidants and phenolic compounds which aid in combating certain cancers. Some of the antioxidants found in this food include flavonoids such as oligomeric proanthocyanidins that protect your cells from free radical damage and prevent the type of dangerous inflammation that may contribute to cancer spread.

6. Source Of Vegetarian Protein

Not only is the food rich in vitamins and minerals, it is also an excellent source of digestible protein for plants. This food contains as much as 14 grams of protein for every 100 grams of serving and 12 separate amino acids to support growth and development of muscles. The protein content is not as high as some beans and legumes, but it is higher than most entire grains.

Cook whole groats with water at a ratio of 1:2 to harness the power of this pseudocereal to yourself, and simmer for 30 minutes or until the grains are tender. For use in pancakes and other breakfast foods as well as your favorite baked goods you can also grind raw groats into flour!

Incorporate buckwheat into your diet:

After soaking and draining the raw groats, people can eat raw buckwheat groats to make them easier to digest. Alternatively, you can boil the groats before adding them groats to salads, sides, or sides.

Breakfast

Buckwheat porridge is another healthful substitute to standard breakfast cereals, or try making pancakes with buckwheat flour, which of course goes well with berries.

Lunch

Buckwheat groats make a superb addition to a salad. Before adding to the salad, you need to boil the buckwheat groats in salted water.

Dinner

Mix the groats with egg to include buckwheat in a stir-fry, then cook them over medium heat for a couple of minutes before adding any other ingredients.

Dessert

Buckwheat muffins are a tasty, gluten-free option for dessert.

Side Effects

Buckwheat can cause a reaction in people suffering from buckwheat allergies. We can experience symptoms when eating buckwheat, such as swelling in the lips, or hives.

2. Capers

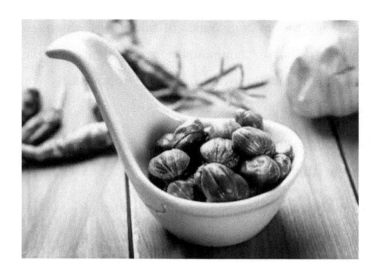

The capers are used primarily for seasoning or garnishing. They are flavor redolent, but they also have many health benefits, surprisingly. They are tangy, spicy and exotic; they add a touch of delight to Italian dishes.

Capers Nutritional Value

Each caper of 100 grams contains 5 grams of carbohydrate, 0.4 grams of sugar, 3 grams of dietary fiber, 0.9 grams of fat, 2 grams of protein, 4 mg of vitamin C, 138 IU vitamin A, 24.6 mg of vitamin K, 0.88 mg of vitamin E, 0.652 mg of niacin, 0.139 mg of riboflavin, 1.7 mg of iron, 2960 mg of sodium, 40 mg of potassium and 96 kJ of energy.

Health Benefits of Capers

1. Antioxidant Powers:

Capers are rich in compounds of flavonoids which include rutin and quercetin. Those compounds are potent antioxidant sources. Antioxidants are known to prevent free radicals which can cause diseases related to cancer and the skin.

Rutin aids in smooth circulation of blood and it is also very helpful in treating strained blood vessels.

Recent research reveals quercetin has analgesic, anti- inflammatory, antibacterial, and anti-carcinogenic properties.

2. Mineral Mine:

Capers comprise minerals like iron, calcium, copper, and high levels of sodium

Calcium aids in building strong bones, and teeth.

Copper combines with some proteins to produce enzymes which act as a catalyst to aid a number of body functions.

Iron aids our muscle to store and use oxygen. It is a part of many enzymes whichaids our body to digest food properly.

3. Vitamin Vitality:

These tasty herbs are storehouses of vitamins such as vitamin A, vitamin K, niacin, and riboflavin (4).

Vitamin A enhances vision and helps us see in the dark. It could also reduce the risk of some cancers. This vital vitamin helps our body to fight off infection and keeps our immune system.

Vitamin K plays a vital role in bone health. It lowers the risk of blood clotting.

Niacin protects against cardiovascular diseases and also helps the nervous and digestive system, the cognitive functions.

Riboflavin, also known as vitamin B2, helps the body turn food into fuel which keeps us healthy. Supporting adrenal activity is also well established. Thus it helps to keep the nervous system safe.

4. Fiberlicious Good:

Capers are powerful fibre sources (5). Fiber cuts down on constipation. A capers table spoon contains 0.3 grams of fiber, about 3 per cent of your daily minimum recommended intake of fiber.

5. Bad Enzyme Buster:

People who include fat and red meat in their daily diet should eat capers, as they destroy certain by-products found in fat-rich meat and foods. Those by-products are often responsible for cardiovascular disease and cancer.

Medicinal Uses of Capers

6. Rheumatism Relief:

In the ancient Greece, capers were used as a treatment for rheumatic pain.

7. Relieves Flatulence:

Caper helps in relieving of stomachache and flatulence. Also, these spicy buds are eaten for improving appetite.

8. Diabetes Buster:

Capers help keep check of diabetes. Capers contain chemicals which control the blood sugar. If you are already using diabetes medicine, avoid consuming high quantities of capers as both tend to lower blood sugar.

9. Congestion Relief:

They are as well known to prevent chest congestion. It reduces phlegm.

Skin Benefits of Capers

10. Dry Skin Relief:

Capers are very good for dry skin. They can be used directly on the skin to keep it moisturized always.

11. Skin Aid:

It is also used to cure skin conditions such as redness in the eye, itching and pimples. Thus capers are used in items for the skin care. Furthermore, because of its antioxidant properties caper helps to slow down the aging process.

Hair Benefits of Capers

12. Promotes Hair Growth:

Since it is rich in vitamin B and magnesium, capers are commonly used in hair care products too. They are both known for fostering hair growth. Vitamin B helps our body circulate in blood. Therefore it supports overall hair health as blood circulation is a primary condition for healthy and shiny hair. Iron helps to avoid loss of hair.

Side Effects of Capers

If you are on a low sodium diet you should avoid capers because they are a rich sodium source.

Extreme thirst is one common sign of eating excess capers. So try taking it in moderate quantities.

Naturally, capers retain water, as they contain a high amount of sodium. This retention of water can therefore make you feel bloated. Be careful to eat excessive quantities of capers.

If you have high blood pressure, then you should avoid eating capers. Sodium excess increases the volume of blood, as it retains water. Excess sodium intake could endanger the body to heart disease.

The risk of developing osteoporosis is another side-effect of eating too much capers. Sodium decreases the density of your bone which causes them to lose strength. It also prevents your body from absorbing calcium which is crucial for bone health building and retaining. Bone weakening also contributes to osteoporosis. And if you have an osteoporosis already, it is better you stay away from capers.

Capers should be strictly avoided when you are pregnant or are undergoing any surgery (12).

Cooking Tips

The capers are used in a variety of sauces, including remoulade or tartare, to bring flavor. When cooked with cheese, they are superb. Understanding the amazing health benefits, you should add them as a salt replacement when frying fish, chicken, turkey, red meat, vegetables and salad. Its tender shoots are used in various dishes, too.

How to Buy Capers?

The dark green ones, in bigger, are the best when it comes to capers. Peppercorn-sized capers from the south of France are considered the world's finest capers.

Storage Tips

Commonly, capers are consumed in brine. Hang these in the refrigerator. You have to make sure they stay submerged in the brine so they don't get dry.

3. Celery

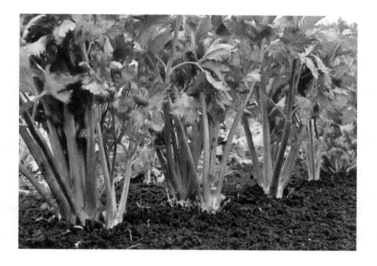

Celery is rich in antioxidants that help remove free radicals from your cells which promote cancer. Celery extract was actually studied for two possible compounds of anticancer: apigenin, and luteolin. Apigenine destroys free radicals in the body and can lead to death in cancer cells. It also seems to be encouraging autophagy, a mechanism in which the body destroys damaged cells or materials that help prevent disease.

Research also suggests luteolin, a celery-based plant flavonoid, could be responsible for its potential anticancer effects. Researchers found in one study that treatment of luteolin decreased tumor levels of the mice by nearly half. And it slowed the tumors remaining to progress. And if that's not enough, China studies suggest that eating two stalks a week could minimize the risk of lung cancer by up to 60%. Some research suggests consuming celery can be effective in treating breast, ovary, pancreas, liver and prostate cancers.

There's no question that adding more vegetables like celery to your diet is a good thing for most of us, however you choose to enjoy them. Celery itself is very nutritious, with many advantages for the body and few downsides. And seeing as adding to a number of recipes is so easy, you may just be promoting it to one of your kitchen staples.

Do not write off celery, whether or not you are involved in eating quarters of celery water. There are many other ways to enjoy this unique vegetable with crunchy stalks, too.

Some of these include:

Chopping it up to use in warm soups

Dicing it for use in an organic tofu scramble

Slicing it thinly for salads and wraps

Chopping it for chickpea salad sandwiches or potato salad

Adding it to stir-fries

Snacking on it raw with almond, peanut, or cashew butter and sprinkling it with raisins or hemp seeds

Adding it to smoothies

4. Chilli

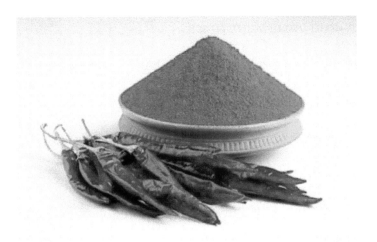

The health benefits documented from hot peppers continue to grow at break-neck speed, similar to the growing popularity of consuming hot foods in different forms. The benefits in terms of heat and safety come from a chemical called capsaicin.

Adding hot peppers, hot sauces and hot powders to food keeps protecting us from food poisoning even though we are now cooling up food. Eating the hottest pepper would magnify those effects to maximize these health benefits.

The health benefits of chillies are infinite.

1. Fight inflammation

Chilli peppers contain a substance called capsaicin which, when eaten, gives peppers their characteristic pungence and produces mild to intense spice. Capsaicin is being studied as an effective treatment for

86

sensory nerve fibre, including arthritis-related pain, psoriasis, and diabetic neuropathy disorders.

2. Natural pain relief

Nowadays topical capsaicin is a common treatment option for discomfort from osteoarthritis. Several review studies of diabetic neuropathy pain management have identified the benefits of topical capsaicin to alleviate the disabling pain associated with this condition.

3. Cardiovascular benefits

Red chilli peppers, such as cayenne, have been shown to decrease blood cholesterol, triglyceride levels, and platelet aggregation, thereby increasing the capacity of the body to absorb fibrin, a material that is essential to blood clot development. Cultures that liberally use hot pepper have a much lower rate of heart attack, stroke and pulmonary embolism.

4. Clear congestion

Not only does capsaicin reduce pain, but its peppery activity also activates secretions that help clear the blocked nose or congested lungs from mucus.

5. Boost immunity

The bright color of red chilli peppers suggests their high beta-carotene or pro-vitamin A content. Only two teaspoons of red chilli peppers provide about six per cent of the daily vitamin C value coupled with more than 10 per cent of the daily vitamin A value. Also referred to as the anti-infection nutrient, vitamin A is necessary for healthy mucous membranes that line the nasal passages, lungs, intestinal tract and urinary tract and function as the body's first line of defense against invading pathogens.

6. Lose weight

Upon eating hot chili peppers all this heat you experience takes energy — and calories to make. Also sweet red peppers have been found to contain substances that increase the thermogenesis (heat production) and oxygen consumption dramatically for more than 20 minutes after feeding.

7. Prevents Bad Breath

Eating hot pepper powder acts as a disinfectant to the air you breathe out by improving the smell of your breath, to keep your significant other attracted to you.

8. Prevents Allergies

Hot peppers can help prevent allergies and hallucinations due to capsaicin's anti-inflammatory effects.

9. Quells Psoriasis

Psoriasis is a itchy skin condition which results in ugly patches of the skin. Capsaicin cream will significantly reduce the number of cells to replicate and help the autoimmune skin lesions to reverse.

5. Chocolate

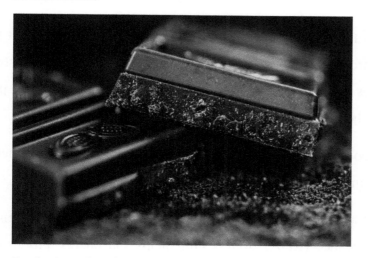

Dark chocolate is rich in minerals, like iron, magnesium, zinc, etc. In dark chocolate, cocoa also contains antioxidants called flavonoids, which can provide several benefits for the health.

What is it that makes dark chocolate deeply desirable? The response is plant phenols-to be precise, cocoa phenols.

Eating dark chocolate will help lower blood pressure if you have moderate high blood pressure, while offset the extra calories by eating less.

Dark chocolate is also loaded with biologically active organic compounds which act as healthy antioxidants. These include amongst others, polyphenols, flavanols, and catechins. Cocoa and dark chocolate contain more antioxidant activity, polyphenols, and flavanols compared to fruits like blueberries and Acai berries.

The high flavonoid levels— potent antioxidants — help protect free radicals from damage to cells and tissues. These radicals are unstable molecules that alter and weaken cells, often resulting from stress, poor diet and the inevitable aging process.

Dark chocolate also contains important amounts of minerals magnesium and copper.

A 1.5-ounce bar contains 15 per cent of magnesium's recommended daily allowance (RDA). Magnesium helps the energy production, strong bones, flexible muscles and powerful nerve propagation. The same bar also includes 34 per cent copper RDA. Copper helps the body develop neurotransmitters and is associated with decreased cardiovascular disease risk.

Since the Mesoamerican civilizations, chocolate and happiness have been combined as a "love food." Chocolate was considered a luxury item and a valuable asset in those early times. For those they cherished, the wealthy made a cocktail of roasted cacao beans with cornmeal, cinnamon, honey and chilies.

Since has science has found an actual chemical bond between chocolate and happiness. Chocolate includes phenylethylamine, a compound that is released into the brain at mental euphoria periods, too. It also contains anandamide, a neurotransmitter for fatty acids which makes you feel more relaxed and less anxious.

The darker that chocolate is, the better. The reason all the accolades are offered by dark chocolate is because it has fewer added sugar and fats than milk or white chocolate. It is higher in beneficial flavonoids, moreover.

Those with the highest share of cacao are better, even when it comes to hot cocoa powder. Choose a bar with at least 70 percent cacao, and just remember— even the deepest of dark chocolates have to be consumed in moderation. There you got it. Science says a dose of dark chocolate every day can be good for your health. No need to wait for a special celebration.

Dark chocolate is a rich source of antioxidants and minerals, and contains less sugar than milk chocolate in general. Some research suggests that dark chocolate can help reduce the risk of heart disease, decrease inflammation and resistance to insulin, and improve brain

91

function. People interested in adding dark chocolate to their diet should bear in mind that fat and calories are high, so moderation is vital.

6. Coffee

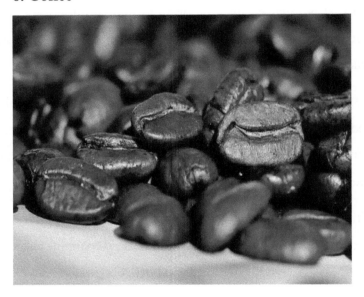

When people think about coffee they usually think about its ability to provide a boost in energy. However, it can also offer some other important health benefits, according to some research, such as a lower risk of liver cancer, type 2 diabetes, and heart failure.

Drinking coffee has advantages for conditions like diabetes, cardiovascular disease, inflammatory bowel disease, and liver disease.

Coffee contains several useful nutrients including riboflavin (vitaminB-2), niacin (vitaminB-3), magnesium, potassium, and various phenolic or antioxidant compounds. Some experts suggest that coffee ingredients such as these and other may benefit the human body in different ways.

How much coffee is safe?

Like so many nutrients and foods too much coffee will cause problems, especially in the digestive tract. But studies have shown that it's safe to drink up to four 8 ounce cups of coffee per day. It shouldn't be hard for coffee drinkers in the US to adhere to those limits, as most drink just a cup of espresso a day.

The potential health benefits

Protection against type 2 diabetes, Parkinson's disease, liver disease, and liver cancer the promotion of a healthy heart

In the sections below, we cover these benefits in more detail.

1. Coffee and diabetes

Coffee can help guard against type 2 diabetes. Those who increased their coffee consumption over 4 years by at least one cup per day had an 11 percent lower type 2 diabetes risk than those who did not increase their intake. A 2017 meta-analysis concluded that people who drank four to six cups of either caffeinated or decaffeinated coffee each day seemed at a lower risk of metabolic syndrome, including type 2 diabetes.

2. Coffee and Parkinson's disease

Various studies have shown that caffeine, contained in coffee and many other drinks, may help protect against Parkinson's illness. One researcher came to the conclusion that people who drink about four cups of coffee a day may have a fivefold lower risk of Parkinson's than those who do not. The caffeine in coffee may also help to control movement in people with Parkinson's.

A 2017 meta-analysis findings suggested a link between coffee consumption and a lower risk of Parkinson's disease, including among people who smoke. This team also found that people who drink coffee may have less probability of experiencing depression and cognitive conditions like Alzheimer's.

There was no evidence to demonstrate that consuming decaffeinated coffee would help prevent Parkinson's disease.

3. Coffee and liver cancer

Italian researchers have found that coffee consumption reduces the risk of hepatic cancer by about 40%. Some of the results suggest that people who drink three cups a day may have a lower risk of 50 per cent. Intake of coffee likely reduces the risk of liver cancer.

4. Coffee and other liver diseases

A 2017 meta-analysis concluded that consuming any type of coffee seemed to reduce the risk of liver cancer, nonalcoholic liver fatty disease, and cirrhosis.

People who consume coffee may also have a lower risk of gallstone disease.

Researchers studied the consumption of coffee among people with primary sclerosing cholangitis (PSC) and primary biliary cirrhosis (PBC) in 2014. Such autoimmune diseases damage the liver's bile ducts.

It was found that people with PSC were more likely to get a lower intake of coffee than those without the disorder. There was no evidence to suggest a difference in coffee intake among people with or without PBC.

In addition, one study in 2014 indicated a correlation between coffee consumption and a lower risk of dying from cirrhosis due to nonviral hepatitis. The researchers proposed that consuming two or more cups of coffee daily could reduce the risk by 66%.

5. Coffee and heart health

One 2012 study concluded that it is possible to protect against heart failure by drinking coffee in moderation, or consuming around two 8-

ounce servings per day. People who drank small amounts of coffee every day had an 11 percent lower heart failure risk compared to those who didn't. One meta-analysis of 2017 found that the consumption of caffeine could have at least a small benefit for cardiovascular health including blood pressure. However, some studies found higher blood lipid (fat) and cholesterol levels in people who were consuming more coffee.

7. Extra Virgin Olive Oil

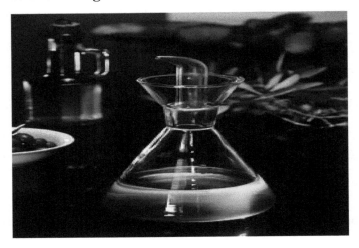

Olive oil is widely acclaimed as one of the healthiest oils in the world. In fact, in regions where olive oil is an essential part of the diet, people tend to live longer and healthier lives.

Extra Virgin Olive Oil (EVOO) is the olive oil of the highest quality possible, harvested from the olive fruit without any heat or chemicals.

1. Extra Virgin Olive Oil is a Fantastic Source of Antioxidants and Healthy Fats

The standard olive oil is distilled and essential nutrients and antioxidants are removed. In comparison, the automatic extraction process used to manufacture Extra Virgin Olive Oil means it preserves all of the olive fruit's nutrients and antioxidants.

Extra Virgin Olive Oil is a rich source of antioxidants and monounsaturated fats, both thought to be cardiovascular health protection.

2. More Olive Oil Could Help Reduce Your Risk of Heart Disease

Extra Virgin Olive Oil contains many active compounds which contribute to the health of the skin. Observational studies consistently find a lower risk of heart disease to those who drink the most.

3. Olive Oil May Protect Against Stroke

Stroke is the second largest killer after heart disease.

It is closely associated with heart disease, which bears many of the same risk factors, such as high cholesterol and high blood pressure. Through observational studies, a diet high through olive has been shown to significantly reduce the risk of strokes.

4. Extra Virgin Olive Oil May Help Lower Your Risk of Type 2 Diabetes

In Australia, about one million people are thought to have type 2 diabetes. Type 2 diabetes is characterized by insulin's decreased potency, the drug that transfers glucose (sugar) out of the blood and into cells to be used for energy. The phenolic compounds found in Extra Virgin Olive Oil are believed to help in glucose metabolism and enhance insulin sensitivity and efficacy.

Extra Virgin Olive Oil can help to improve the absorption of insulin, which can help protect against type 2 diabetes or the pre-existing diabetes.

5. Extra Virgin Olive Oil is the Best Cooking Oil

Many different cooking oils claim to be the best.

However, considering the major factors affecting how oil reacts to high temperatures–oxidative stability and monounsaturated fat ratio– Extra Virgin Olive Oil is number one. Extra Virgin Olive Oil is easily the best choice for cooking if you consider its oxidative stability, superior antioxidant content and ratio of monounsaturated fat, as well as its diverse flavor profile.

6. Cooking With Extra Virgin Olive Oil Can Make Your Food More Nutritious

Cooking with Extra Virgin Olive Oil may help retain the amount of nutrients and antioxidants in the cooked food that would otherwise be lost or damaged, and may in some cases increase.

7. Olive Oil Consumption May Improve Bone Health

Olive oil, especially polyphenol-rich ones such as Extra Virgin Olive Oil, can prevent bone loss with ageing. Emerging evidence links the consumption of polyphenols and olive oil to a reduced risk of bone loss in older years. This needs more work to confirm this with any confidence.

8. The Compounds in Olive Oil May Protect Against Certain Cancers

It's known what and how we eat will affect the risk of cancer. Observational studies have shown a lower incidence of certain cancers in regions where intake of olive oil is high. Extra virgin olive oil could possibly, at least theoretically, defend against certain cancers.

9. A Diet High in Extra Virgin Olive Oil May be Good for Brain Health

Olive oil may theoretically reduce the risk of Alzheimer's disease and dementia associated with aging. Extra Virgin Olive Oil's phenolic ingredients may help clear off the chemicals that cause brain degeneration. Early research indicates that the substances responsible for Alzheimer's disease and dementia may be reduced by a diet high in extra virgin olive oil.

10. Olive Oil Can Contribute to Health and Longevity

Consistently, observational studies suggest that those who eat a diet high in extra virgin olive oil tend to live longer.

8. Green Tea – ideally matcha

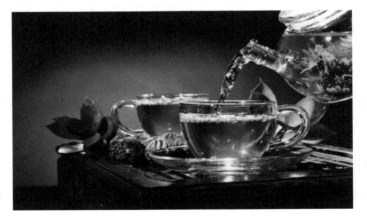

There is that awareness that daily consumption of Japanese green tea, and particularly matcha, will support your health and overall well-being enormously.

In fact, the reason matcha has amazing health benefits is because you are eating the whole crop. In comparison, you only get about 10 per cent of the nutrients from the tea leaves when you drink steeped green tea. That's right, some 90 per cent of the health benefits of green tea in the tea pot are left behind. And then, what do you do? Throw it away!

So to capture the mostbenefits of a green tea, just try to drink matcha every day.

l	Lowered Cholesterol	Lowered
lism	& Blood-Pressure	Blood Sugar
Calories	*Reducing Risk of*	
g Fat	*Heart-Disease*	
Weight-Loss	*& Stroke*	*Relief from Diabetes*

hibited Cancer	Protection Against	Strengthening
ll Growth	Pneumonia	Skin Cells
east Cancer	*Combats Viral Disease*	*Anti-Ageing*
ng Cancer		

ATCHA HEALTH BENEFITS

In fact, the benefits of green tea for particular teas are greatly increased by shading the tea plant a few weeks before harvest time. Shading slows the leaf's growth, causing the nutrients to swell, and adding features like UMAMI and sweetness. That's just one explanation why green Japanese tea is the healthiest of all teas! Matcha, Hon Gyokoro and Kabusecha have the most antioxidants and provide the green tea with the most health benefits as they are shaded in this manner.

Moreover, how does Matcha help me to lose weight?

Here, the key word is' help.' If you are already following a weight-loss program then matcha can certainly help by providing you with higher energy levels without the need to consume more calories (matcha is almost calorie-free, but of course not matcha latte!). And it can actually help to burn fat, without raising levels of blood pressure, heart rate or sugar. It's a natural product so there's no worry about allergic reactions or other problems that some people experience with alternative dietary supplements or energy bars and beverages.

Moreover, Don't Forget The Most Important Thing About Matcha...

Matcha is one of Japanese tea's highest grades and is served in a micro-ground powdered form, so you're literally drinking the whole leaf while you drink it! That's why in just one serving of matcha there is about 10 times the nutritional value, compared to over 10 cups of other steeped green teas. The benefits of matcha tea are x10!

9. Kale

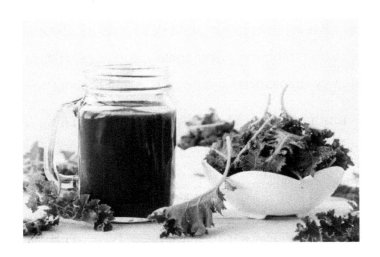

Kale is a nutrient rich, green, leafy, cruciferous vegetable. It can bring a range of health benefits to the entire body.

Kale contains fibre, antioxidants, calcium, vitamins C and K, iron, and a wide variety of other nutrients that can help prevent various health issues. Antioxidants help the body eliminate undesirable toxins resulting from natural processes and environmental pressures.

There are many potent antioxidants present in kale, including quercetin and kaempferol, which have many beneficial health effects. Kale is exceptionally high in vitamin C, an antioxidant which has a lot of important body functions. Indeed a single cup of raw kale provides more vitamin C than an orange.

Kale contains substances that bind bile acids and decrease body cholesterol levels. Specifically Steamed kale is successful. Vitamin K

104

is an essential vitamin involved in clotting the blood. A single cup of kale produces vitamin K 7 times the RDA.

Throughout test-tube and animal studies, Kale contains compounds that have been shown to help fight cancer but the medical data is conflicting. Kale is very rich in beta-carotene, an antioxidant which can be converted into vitamin A by the body.

Kale contains many essential minerals, some of which are generally lacking in the modern diet. These include magnesium, calcium and potassium.

Kale is rich in lutein and zeaxanthin, nutrients associated with a significantly reduced risk of macular degeneration and cataracts.

Kale is a nutrient-dense, low-calorie food that makes an excellent addition to a diet for weight loss.

Nutrition

The following table indicates the quantity of each element in a cup of boiled kale, weighing about 118 grams (g) without adding salt.

It also shows how much each nutrient needs an adult according to the Americans ' Dietary Guidelines 2015–2020. Requirements vary according to sex and age of the individual.

Nutrient	Amount in 1 cup	Daily adult requirement
Energy (calories)	42.5	1,800–3,000
Carbohydrate in grams (g)	6.3, including 1.4 g of sugar	130
Fiber (g)	4.7	22.4–33.6
Protein (g)	3.5	46–56
Calcium in milligrams (mg)	177	1,000–1,200
Iron (mg)	1.0	8–18
Magnesium (mg)	29.5	320–420
Phosphorus (mg)	49.6	700
Potassium (mg)	170	4,700
Sodium (mg)	18.9	2,300
Zinc (mg)	0.3	8–11
Copper (mg)	0.8	900

Manganese (mg)	0.6	1.8–2.3
Selenium in micrograms (mcg)	1.1	55
Vitamin C (mg)	21	75–90
Folate (mcg DFE)	76.7	400
Betaine (mg)	0.4	No data
Beta carotene (mcg)	2,040	No data
Lutein + zeaxanthin (mcg)	5,880	No data
Vitamin E (mg)	1.9	15
Vitamin K (mcg)	494	90–120
Vitamin A (mcg RAE)	172	700–900

Kale also contains a number of antioxidants and B vitamins. Fortunately, supplementing your diet with kale is relatively simple. You can just add it to your salads, or use it in your recipes.

A popular snack is kale chips, where you drizzle over your kale some extra virgin olive oil or avocado oil, add some salt, and then bake an oven until it's dry. It tastes delicious, and makes a great snack that is crunchy, super healthy. There are also many people who add kale to their smoothies to boost the nutritional value.

Kale is surely one of the healthiest and most nutritious foods on the planet at the end of the day. If you want to boost the amount of nutrients you are taking in dramatically, consider loading up on kale.

10. Lovage

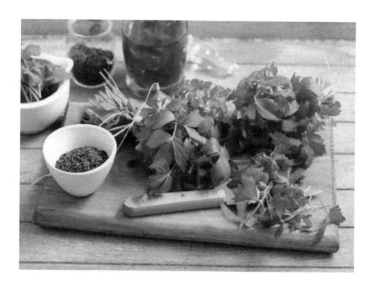

Lovage is a perennial, easy to grow plant due to its hardy properties. It belongs to the same family as dill, parsley, and carrots. The Lovage plant's dark green leaves resemble cilantro and Italian parsley in shape and colour, and their stalks are often compared with celery stalks (in appearance, and to a lesser extent, in flavour). Lovage has a very strong smell, and a moist and herbal flavor.

The most commonly used parts of the Lovage plant for medicinal purposes include its leaves, branches, and roots. Lovage is widely converted into an essential oil and may be used in infusions, tinctures, decoctions (preparations produced by boiling fresh or dried herbs in water to remove water-soluble ingredients), vinegars, elixirs, and lozenges.

Lovage, a rare medicinal plant, can be consumed as a fresh vegetable or fried to improve the taste and add nutrients to the dish. Its claimed benefits include enhancing urinary health and providing antibacterial properties.

Health Benefits

This means that the herb can stimulate urination (and help flush the bladder and kidneys by increasing urine output) without loss of vital electrolytes (such as sodium).

The plant is also thought to contain a calming agent called eucalyptol which may help to reduce lung irritation and promote healing of certain forms of respiratory disorders (such as pleurisy).

Medical Uses

Although clinical research data are insufficient to support most of the claims about the health benefits of lovage, the plant has traditionally been used to treat many health conditions, which includes:

Stomach disorders

Cough and respiratory conditions (such as pleurisy)

Fever

Sore throat

Colic (in young children)

Gas

Rheumatism/arthritis

Urinary tract infections

Kidney stones

Gout

Boils

Malaria

Migraines

Jaundice

The findings of the preliminary study confirm some of the herbal supplement's reported health benefits, such as reproductive safety and antibacterial properties, among others:

A diuretic effect

A carminative action

An expectorant effect (helping to loosen phlegm)

An antibacterial effect

An anti-inflammatory effect

111

A stimulant effect

An appetite stimulant effect

A diaphoretic action (to stimulate perspiration and help reduce fevers)

An emmenagogue (helping to regulate menstruation)

11. Medjool Dates

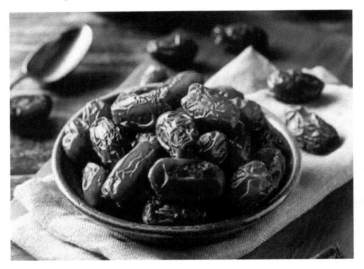

All evidence points to the fact that you have to avoid sugary foods to improve your health. Studies show that eating refined sugar causes depletion of energy, also known as the dreaded "sugar crash" when empty calories use the vitamins and minerals in our body to turn it into fuel. Think of it to your body like a credit card. Rather than using your healthcare building resources, refined sugar uses your resources and creates a deficit!

The good news is that nature, in very sweet packages, gives us incredible nutrition. While satisfying your sweet tooth, dates provide the nutrients you need.

1. Dates are a source of antioxidants. All dates, whether fresh or dried, have different antioxidant types. Fresh dates contain anthocyanidins and carotenoids, while dried dates, like green tea, contain polyphenols. Khalas (aka Madina) dates are the highest in antioxidants compared with varieties of other dates.

2. Dates can be good for blood sugar balance. Researchers on diabetes have demonstrated that the dates have low glycemic impact. It means eating dates individually, or with a meal, will help people with type 2 diabetes control blood sugar and fat levels in their body.

3. Dates can help reduce blood pressure.A standard 5-or6-date serving provides around 80 milligrams of magnesium, an essential mineral that helps dilate blood vessels. Research shows that magnesium supplementation can reduce blood pressure by 370 milligrams. Dates are a delicious way of softening your magnesium intake.

4. Dates contain a brain booster. Every small date includes more than two milligrams of choline, the memory neurotransmitter, a B vitamin that's a factor of acetylcholine. Higher intake of choline is associated with better memory and learning making it a key nutrient at risk for Alzheimer's children and older adults.

5. Dates help maintain bone mass. Bone loss can be reduced in post-menopause women with osteopenia by increasing potassium intake. One dried date provides almost 140 milligrams of that precious nutrient. High intake of potassium protects bone mass by reducing the quantity of calcium excreted through the renals.

12. Parsley

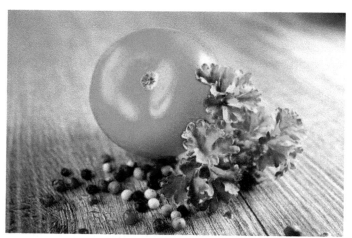

114

Impressive health benefits and uses of parsley.

Reduce the risk of getting cancer. Eating parsley can reduce the risk of breast, digestive tract, skin and prostate cancers.

Enhance immune function. Petersilage can help to modulate the immune system.

Beat inflammation.

Fight disease.

Protect your blood vessels.

Parsley is a low-calorie, herb dense in nutrients. It is especially rich in vitamins K, A and C. Parsley provides several strong antioxidants that may help prevent damage to the cells and reduce your risk of certain diseases. Perseys are rich in vitamin K, an essential nutrient for optimal bone health. Eating foods high in this nutrient was associated with a reduced risk of fractures and improved mineral density in the bone. Parsley contains various antioxidants— such as flavonoids and vitamin C— that can be of benefit to the fight against cancer. Parsley contains lutein, zeaxanthin and beta-carotene, plant compounds that protect the health of the eyes and can reduce your risk of certain age-related eye conditions such as AMD. Pereza is rich in folate, a B vitamin that protects your heart and can reduce your heart disease risk.

It has been shown that the parsley extract has antibacterial properties in test tube studies. However more research is needed.

Parsley may be used as dried spice or as a fresh herb. Typically dried flakes are added to hot dishes such as soup and spaghetti, while the fresh herb is an excellent addition to salads and dressings.

Parsley is a flexible herb which provides concentrated nutrient supply. It is especially rich in vitamins A, C and K. Within parsley, the vitamins and beneficial plant compounds can enhance bone health, guard against chronic diseases and provide antioxidant advantages. Dried or fresh leaves can be easily incorporated into your diet by adding them to soups, salads, marinades, and sauces.

13. Red Chicory

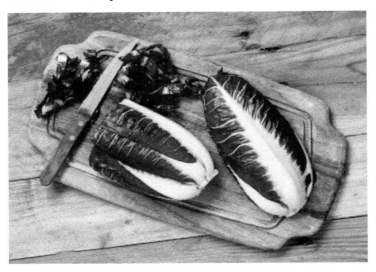

116

Radicchio is a type of leafy chicory with dark reddish-purple leaves and white veins, also known as Cichoriumintybus and Italian chicory.

Radicchio, though widely mistaken for red cabbage or lettuce, has a distinctly bitter taste that goes well with many Italian dishes. It is a traditional Mediterranean diet ingredient which emphasizes whole plant foods. You may wonder how different radicchio is from other more traditional leafy vegetables such as cabbage and lettuce, and if it's worth adding to your diet.

Radicchio is a bitter chicory variety which is widely used in Italian dishes. Radicchio is rich in zinc, copper and vitamin K while low in calories.

Health benefits

Cichoriumintybus's traditional therapeutic applications include wound healing as well as diarrhea care, heart health preservation, and blood sugar control. Radicchio provides potential health benefits, primarily because of strong plant compounds.

Other potential health benefits

Radicchio compounds may offer other health benefits but more research is needed to identify specific applications and doses:

May promote strong bones. Radicchio contains a large amount of vitamin K that regulates and promotes your body's calcium accumulation, and supports bone strength.

May support blood sugar control. Adults who consumed 1.25 cups (300 ml) of a normal4-week chicory root extract drink had decreased levels of hemoglobin A1c, an indication of long-term blood sugar levels (15Trusted Source).

May improve digestive health. In the same study, during consumption of chicory root extract, participants reported an improvement in bowel regularity. This may be due to its content of inulin fibre, which is important for gastrointestinal health.

14. Red Onions

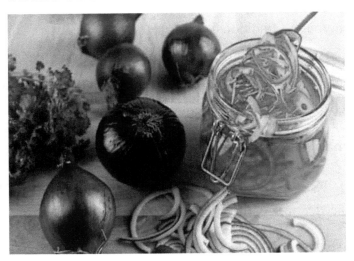

118

Even though all vegetables are important to health, there are certain types that offer unique benefits.

These vegetables contain various vitamins, minerals, and potent plant compounds which have been demonstrated in many ways to promote health. In fact, onions ' medicinal properties have been recognized since ancient times, when used to treat ailments such as headaches, heart disease, and mouth sores. Onions are low in calories and yet rich in nutrients, including vitamin C, vitamins B and potassium. Eating onions can help to reduce risk factors for heart disease, such as high blood pressure, increased levels of triglycerides and inflammation. Red onions are high in anthocyanins that can guard against heart disease, other tumors, and diabetes. A diet that is rich in allium vegetables such as onions can have a protective effect against some cancer. Consuming them can help reduce high blood sugar, thanks to the many beneficial compounds found in onions. Consumption of onion is correlated with increased mineral density in the body. Onions have proven to inhibit the growth of potentially harmful bacteria such as E. Coli, S. Aurora. Onions are a rich source of probiotic drugs that help enhance digestive health, strengthen your gut's bacterial balance and protect your immune system. It is easy to add onions to the savory dishes, including bacon, guacamole, meat dishes, soups, and baked products.

The health benefits are quite impressive in relation to onions. Such nutrient-packed vegetables contain potent compounds that can reduce the heart disease risk and some cancers. Oignons have antibacterial properties and promote digestive health which can improve immune function. What's more, they are versatile and can be used to increase any savory dish's flavour. An easy way to benefit your overall health is to add more onions to your diet.

15. Red Wine

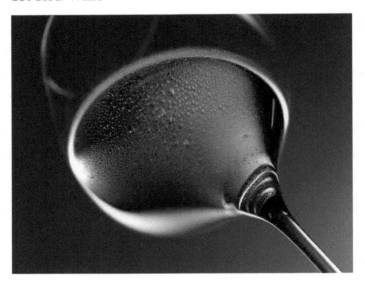

Red wine contains resveratrol, but it may not be the safest way to consume it, because alcohol intake carries with it dangers of its own.

Gut microbiome and cardiovascular health.

Raising levels of omega-3 fatty acids.

Heart health and type-2 diabetes.

Healthy blood vessels and blood pressure.

Brain damage after stroke.

16. Rocket

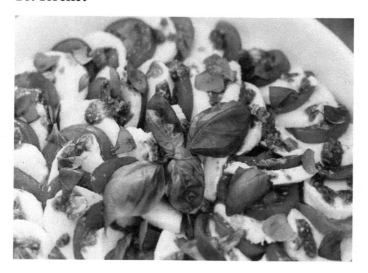

It is also called arugula and contains numerous nutrients. These include vitamin C, K and A and high nitrate levels. ...

Protect against cancer. ...

Vitamin K for a healthy heart, bones, and skin.

Boost eyesight with rocket.

17. Soy

121

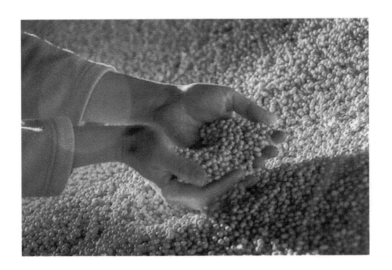

Soybeans have high protein content and are a decent source of both carbs and fat. They are a rich source of diverse vitamins, minerals and beneficial compounds for plants, such as isoflavones. For this reason regular intake of soybean can alleviate menopause symptoms and reduce your risk of prostate and breast cancer.

What are the health benefits of soya?

The key benefits of soya are its high protein content, nutrients, vitamins and insoluble fibre.

The high fiber content makes valuable soya beans and other foods containing soya in cases of constipation, high cholesterol and type-2 diabetes.

18. Strawberries

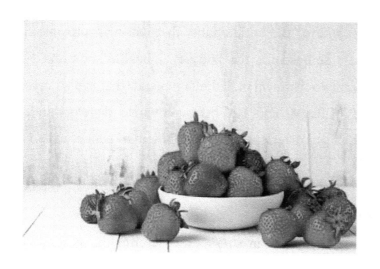

Strawberries are soft, juicy and light red. These are an excellent source of manganese and vitamin C, and also contain decent amounts of folate (vitamin B9) and potassium. Strawberries are very high in antioxidants and plant compounds which may aid heart health and regulation of blood sugar. You should be, if you are not already a lover of strawberries. These are not only sweet, summery and tasty but also a bona fide superfood. The advantages of strawberries are limitless, nutrient-rich and filled with antioxidants (like vitamin C), and some will even impress you.

Benefits

1. Maintain your healthy vision

2. Give your immunity a boost

3. Ward off cancer

Vitamin C is one of the antioxidants that can help prevent cancer, since the best defense for the body is a healthy immune system. Another is a phytochemical called ellagic acid, that is also present in strawberries. "Ellagic acid has been shown to develop anticancer properties such as preventing the development of cancer cells.

4. Keep your wrinkles at bay

The power of vitamin C in strawberries continues, as it is vital to collagen production, which helps to improve the elasticity and resilience of skin. Since we lose collagen as we age, eating vitamin C-rich foods can lead to healthier, younger looking skin. But vitamin C is not the only natural wrinkle fighter found in that fruit.

Lower your cholesterol

Cardiac disease is one of the leading causes of death among Canadian women, according to the Heart and Stroke Foundation. Fortunately, strawberries ' benefits include powerful heart-healthy boosters.

Reduce pesky inflammation

The antioxidants and phytochemicals present in strawberries can also help to reduce joint inflammation which can lead to arthritis and heart disease.

Regulate your blood pressure

Boost your fibre intake

Fibre is a must for safe digestion and strawberries usually produce about 2 g of weight management aid per serving.

One of the best defenses against type 2 diabetes and heart disease is maintaining a healthy weight, not to mention just being good for your overall wellbeing.

Help to promote pre-natal health

Folate is a prescribed B-vitamin for pregnant women or those who are trying to conceive, and strawberries are a good source of 21 mg per meal.

19. Turmeric

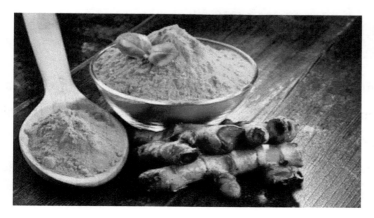

Turmeric Contains Bioactive Compounds With Powerful Medicinal Properties. ...

Curcumin Is a Natural Anti-Inflammatory Compound. ...

Turmeric Dramatically Increases the Antioxidant Capacity of the Body. ...

Curcumin increases the neurotrophic factor derived from the intestine, related to better brain function and lower brain disease risk.

20. Walnut

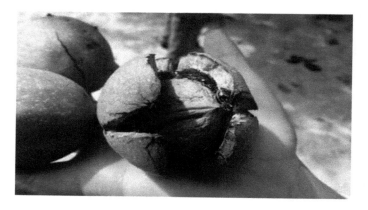

A handful of walnuts contain nearly twice as much antioxidant as an equivalent of any other commonly consumed nut, "US chemistry professor and study researcher Joe Vinson said in a statement." But unfortunately, people don't eat a lot of them. "His advice: eat seven walnuts a day.

What are the benefits of eating walnuts?

126

Rich in Antioxidants.

Super Plant Source of Omega-3s.

May Decrease Inflammation.

Promotes a Healthy Gut.

May Reduce Risk of Some Cancers.

Supports Weight Control.

May Help Manage Type 2 Diabetes and Lower Your Risk.

May Help Lower Blood Pressure.

Chapter 5
The Sirtfood Diet Phases

Such unique foods function by activating specific proteins such as sirtuins in the body. Sirtuins are thought to prevent the body's cells from dying when under stress, and are thought to control inflammation, metabolism, and aging processes. Scientists also conclude that sirtuins affect the body's ability to burn fat and improve metabolism, contributing to a weight loss of seven pounds a week while retaining muscle.

The Sirtfood Diet has two phases that last three weeks overall. You can then proceed to "sirtify" your diet by including as many sirt foods as possible into your meals.

The actual recipes for these two phases can be found in the book The Sirtfood Diet, which was published by founders of the diet. You'll need to do it to keep up with the diet.

The meals are full of sirtfoods but in addition to the "top 20 sirtfoods," other ingredients do.

Most of the ingredients and sirtfoods are easy to find.

Three of the signature ingredients needed for these two phases—matcha green tea powder, lovage, and buckwheat — can, however, be costly or hard to find.

A large part of the diet is its green juice, which you'll have to make between one and three times a day. A juicer (a mixer won't work) and a kitchen scale will be required, as the ingredients are described by weight. The recipe is below:

Sirtfood Green Juice

75 grams (2.5 oz) kale

30 grams (1 oz) arugula (rocket)

5 grams parsley

2 celery sticks

1 cm (0.5 in) ginger

Half a green apple

Half a lemon

Half a teaspoon matcha green tea

Juice all ingredients together, except the green tea powder and lemon, and pour them into a bottle. Juice the lemon by hand, then whisk in both the lemon juice and the green tea powder.

Phase One

The first process lasts for seven days, with calorie restriction and lots of green juice involved. It's meant to boost your weight loss and promise to help you lose 7 pounds (3.2 kg) in seven days.

Intake of calories during the first three days of phase one is reduced to 1,000 calories. You drink three green drinks, plus one dinner, per day. You can choose from recipes in the book every day, all of which include sirtfood as a big part of the meal.

Highlights of meals include miso-glazed tofu, the omelet sirtfood or a shrimp stir-fry with buckwheat noodles.

Calorie intake is raised to 1,500 on days, from Phase One 4–7. It involves two green juices a day and two more sirtfood-rich meals that can be picked from the book.

Phase Two

Phase 2, which lasts two weeks. You will begin to loose weight slowly during this "maintenance" period.

This phase has no clear calorie limit. Alternatively, you enjoy three sirt-fed meals and one green juice a day. The meals are again taken from the recipes included in the book.

After the Diet

Those two stages may be repeated as often as you wish for further weight loss.

However, upon finishing those stages, you are advised to start "sirtifying" your diet by consistently integrating sirt foods into your meals.

There are a number of Sirtfood Diet books, full of sirtfood rich recipes. You can also include sirt foods as a snack in your diet, or in recipes that you already have.

You are further encouraged to continue consuming the green juice everyday.

Thus the Sirtfood Diet becomes more a change in lifestyle than a one-time diet.

Chapter 6
Sirtfood Diet plan

You limit your intake to 1000 calories per day for the first week, which involves eating three sirtfood green juices and one sirtfood rich meal a day. You increase your diet to 1500 calories a day the next week, and eat two sirt-rich meals and two green juices. However, there's no set plan in the long run, it's all about changing your diet to include as many sirt foods as you can, which should make you feel better and more energized.

Sirtfood Recipes

If you're thinking about trying the Sirtfood diet, this book is here to motivate you with five delicious recipes for a 7-day program to lose an average of 7 lb, while adding Sirtfood recipes to your diet can help if you'd like a more relaxed approach.

The Sirtfood Juice

A good way to get going is with The Sirtfood Juice–so I've put this in the recipe to start you off as an extra bonus. The book recommends that you drink 3 juices and add 1 meal for the first 3 days, then 2 juices and 2 meals for the next 4.Sirtfood Green Juice (serves 1)

Ingredients:

2 large handfuls (75g) kale

A large handful (30g) rocket

A very small handful (5g) flat-leaf parsley

A very small handful (5g) lovage leaves (optional)

2–3 large stalks (150g) green celery, including its leaves

½ medium green apple

Juice of ½ lemon

½ level tsp matcha green tea

Instructions:

Bring together the greens (kale, rocket, parsley and lovage, if used), and sauté them. We consider juicers can really vary in their performance when juicing leafy vegetables and before going on to the other ingredients, you may need to re-juice the remains. The goal is to finish off the greens with around 50ml of water.

Now you can peel the lemon and also bring it through the juicer, but we find it much easier to just pinch the lemon in the juice by hand. You should have about 250ml of juice in total by this point, maybe a little bit more. It's only when the juice is blended and ready to serve that you add the green tea matcha.

In a glass, pour a small amount of juice, then add the matcha, and stir vigorously with a fork or tablespoon. In the first two drinks of the day, we only use matcha, because it contains small amounts of caffeine

133

(the same quality as a regular tea cup). When drank late. Once the matcha is diluted add the remainder of the drink, it may keep them awake for those not used to it.

Give it a swirl end, and the juice is ready to drink. Easy to top up with plain water, as you like.

Sirt Muesli (serves 1)

Simply mix the dry ingredients and place them in an airtight container if you want to make this in bulk or cook it the night before. The next day all you need to do is add the strawberries and yoghurt and it's ready to go.

Ingredients:

20g buckwheat flakes

10g buckwheat puffs

15g coconut flakes or desiccated coconut

40g Medjool dates, pitted and chopped

15g walnuts, chopped

10g cocoa nibs

100g strawberries, hulled and chopped

100g plain Greek yoghurt (or vegan alternative, such as soya or coconut yoghurt)

Instructions:

Mix (leave out the strawberries and yoghurt if not serving straight away).

Aromatic breast of chicken with red and kale onions and tomato and chili salsa (serves 1)

Ingredients:

120g skinless, boneless chicken breast

2 tsp ground turmeric

Juice of ¼ lemon

1 tbsp extra virgin olive oil

50g kale, chopped

20g red onion, sliced

1 tsp chopped fresh ginger

50g buckwheat

For the salsa

130g tomato (about 1)

1 bird's eye chilli, finely chopped

1 tbsp capers, finely chopped 5g parsley, finely chopped

Juice of ¼ lemon

Instructions:

Cut the eye from the tomato to make the sauce, then slice it very good, making care to keep as much of the liquid as possible. Mix with the chilli, capers, lemon juice and parsley. You might put it all in a blender but the end result is a bit different.

Heat the oven to 220oC / gas 7. Marinate the chicken breast with the turmeric, lemon juice and a little oil in 1 tablespoon. Heat an ovenproof frying pan until hot, then add the marinated chicken and cook on each side for about a minute or so until pale yellow, then move to the oven (place on a baking tray if your pan is not ovenproof) for 8-10 minutes or until cooked through. Clear from the oven, cover with foil and allow to cool before serving for 5 minutes.

Alternatively, simmer the kale for 5 minutes in a steamer. In a little butter, fried the red onions and ginger until soft but not flavored, then add the cooked kale and fry for another minute. Fry the buckwheat with the remaining turmeric tablespoon in compliance with the package directions. Serve with chicken, tomatoes, and salsa.

Sirtfood bites (makes 15-20 bites)

Ingredients:

120g walnuts

30g dark chocolate (85 per cent cocoa solids), broken into pieces; or cocoa nibs

250g Medjool dates, pitted

1 tbsp cocoa powder

1 tbsp ground turmeric

1 tbsp extra virgin olive oil

The scraped seeds of 1 vanilla pod or 1 tsp vanilla extract

1–2 tbsp water

Instructions:

Place the walnuts and chocolate in a food processor and grind them until the powder is perfect.

Add all the remaining ingredients except water and mix until the mixture forms a ball. Based on the consistency of the paste, you may or may not have to apply the water-you don't want it to be too wet.

Shape the mixture into bite-sized balls using your hands, then refrigerate for at least 1 hour in an airtight container before eating them. In some more chocolate or desiccated coconut you could roll some of the balls to create a different texture, if you like. We should keep it in your fridge for up to 1 week.

Asian king prawn stir-fry with buckwheat noodles (serves 1)

Ingredients:

150g shelled raw king prawns, deveined

2 tsp tamari (you can use soy sauce if you are not avoiding gluten)

2 tsp extra virgin olive oil

75g soba (buckwheat noodles)

1 garlic clove, finely chopped

1 bird's eye chilli, finely chopped

1 tsp finely chopped fresh ginger

20g red onions, sliced

40g celery, trimmed and sliced

75g green beans, chopped

50g kale, roughly chopped

100ml chicken stock

5g lovage or celery leaves

Instructions:

Heat a frying pan over high heat, then cook the prawns for 2–3 minutes in 1 tablespoon of the tamari and 1 teaspoon of butter. Place the prawns onto a tray. Wipe the pan out with paper from the oven, as you will be using it again.

Cook the noodles 5–8 minutes in boiling water, or as indicated on the package. Drain and set aside.

While, over medium - high heat, fry the garlic, chilli and ginger, red onion, celery, beans and kale in the remaining oil for 2–3 minutes. Remove the stock and bring to the boil, then simmer for one to two minutes until the vegetables are cooked but crunchy.

Add the prawns, noodles and leaves of lovage / celery to the pan, bring back to the simmer, then reduce the heat and drink.

Strawberry buckwheat tabouleh

Ingredients:

50g buckwheat

1 tbsp ground turmeric

80g avocado

65g tomato

20g red onion

25g Medjool dates, pitted

1 tbsp capers

30g parsley

100g strawberries, hulled

1 tbsp extra virgin olive oil

Juice of ½ lemon

30g rocket

Instructions:

Cook the buckwheat with the turmeric as indicated on the package. Drain to cool and leave on one side.

Chop the avocado, basil, red onion, dates, capers and parsley thinly and mix with the fresh buckwheat. Slice the strawberries, then mix the oil and lemon juice softly into the salad. Serve on a bed of rocket.

How Is It Effective?

The Sirtfood Diet's authors make bold claims, including that the diet can induce super-charge weight loss, turn on your "skinny gene" and prevent disease.

The problem here is that there isn't enough proof to back them.

There is no compelling evidence to date that the Sirtfood Diet has a more positive effect on weight loss than any other diet controlled by calories.

And although many of those foods have healthful properties, no long-term human studies have been conducted to assess if eating a diet rich in sirt foods has any measurable health benefits.

Nonetheless, a pilot study carried out by the authors and involving 39 participants from their fitness center is recorded in the Sirtfood Diet book. Nevertheless, the results of this study do not seem to have been published elsewhere.

Participants followed the diet for a week and were exercising daily. Participants lost an average of 7 pounds (3.2 kg) at the end of the week, and retained or even added muscle mass.

These findings, though, are hardly unexpected. Limiting your calorie intake to 1,000 calories, and actively exercising, will almost always cause weight loss.

However, this kind of rapid weight loss is neither real nor long-lasting, and after the first week, this study did not follow participants to see if they gained any of the weight back, which is usually so.

As well as consuming fat and muscle, when the body is drained of energy, it uses the emergency energy stores, or glycogen.

That glycogen molecule requires 3–4 water molecules for storage. If the body uses glycogen, the water always gets rid of it. It's known as "water weight."

Only about one-third of the weight loss comes from fat during the first week of severe calorie restriction while the other two-thirds come from skin, muscle, and glycogen. The body must replenish its glycogen stores as soon as the calorie intake rises, and the weight comes right back.

Unfortunately, this form of calorie restriction can also cause your body to decrease its metabolic rate, allowing energy requirements to be even lower in calories per day. This diet is likely to help you lose a few pounds in the beginning, but it'll probably return as soon as the diet is over.

As far as disease prevention is concerned, it is certainly three weeks not long enough to have any meaningful long-term effects. On the other hand, it may very well be a smart idea to add sirtfood to your regular diet over the long term. You might as well miss the detox in that scenario, so start doing it now.

Is It Healthy and Sustainable?

Sirtfoods are almost always healthy choices, and thanks to their antioxidant or anti-inflammatory effects, they can even provide certain health benefits.

But consuming only a handful of particularly healthy foods can not meet all the nutritional needs of your body.

The Sirtfood Diet is unnecessarily restrictive and does not offer any simple, special health benefits over any other diet.

Furthermore, eating just 1,000 calories is not typically recommended without a doctor's supervision. For many people, only eating 1,500 calories per day is overly restrictive.

In fact, the diet includes up to three green drinks per day. While juices can be a good source of vitamins and minerals, they are also a source of sugar and contain almost none of the nutritious fibers that whole fruits and vegetables do (13).

What's more, sipping on fruit all day long is a bad idea for both blood sugar and teeth (14Trusted Source).

Not to mention, because the diet is so limited in calories and food choice, protein, vitamins, and minerals are more than likely insufficient, particularly during the first process.

This diet can be difficult to stick to for the whole three weeks due to the low calorie levels and limited food choices.

Chapter 7
A Complete Week Plan On Sirtfoods

The truth behind the seven-day eating plan that claims to strip away weight. The diet promises to torch fat within a week, while leaving intact muscle. But there's more to Sirtfoods than miraculous promises–if the evidence behind it is working out, it might show that we've been talking about eating healthy the wrong way for decades.

One way or another, you've heard of the Sirt Diet, even if you don't recognize the name. It is described as the kilo-shredding program in news reports that encourages you to eat chocolate and drink red wine, pledging to look like a supermodel and behave like a superhero.

But the fact is, behind Sirt there is much more analytical clout than the usual drop-fat-fast scheme. It is based on a family of compounds which have only been found in the past decade, and experimental evidence shows that they are much more significant than previously thought. And if the people behind it are right, then when we're talking about what to eat we need to change our attention.

What's the truth? What's the evidence? And what's the science behind it all?

Science first. Sirtuins–from which Sirt gets its name–are a group of Silent Information Regulator (SIR) proteins that ramp up our metabolism, increase muscle performance, turn on processes of fat burning, minimize inflammation and repair cell damage. In short, sirtuins make us fitter, leaner and safer (there's also proof that they might help fight serious diseases like Alzheimer's and diabetes –more on that later).

145

Mild sources of stress–including exercise and calorie restriction–cause the development of sirtuins by the body, but it has been discovered recently that chemical compounds known as sirtuin activators, naturally present in fruit and vegetables, can do the same. Many products–syrtfoods, as diet founders Aidan Goggins and Glen Matten called them –are particularly high in these sirtuin activators and so, the theory goes, if you eat a diet mainly made of those foods you will lose fat and improve your health.

Goggins and Matten developed the Sirt Diet to test this idea, the seven-day eating plan that triggered all the fuss. It's clear enough: the daily calorie consumption is reduced to 1,000 during the first three days and comprises of three green juices, with a Sirtfood-rich lunch. Calorie intake is raised to 1,500 on the fourth to seventh day, which consists of two drinks and two meals. The advice after that all-out first week is to eat a balanced diet high in Sirtfoods, along with more green juices. Which sounds awful on the face of it: even the most strict diets qualify for more calories. But is it?

The juice is key: it is like fuel from rockets. Following the initial week, there was plain sailing during the diet and after three weeks, I was 5 kg lighter. Yet, crucially, I looked the happiest I had in a couple years as well. I reduced my body fat, I ate well, I didn't have any problems in my stomach and I felt energized... I taught and practiced half a dozen lessons a week with great recovery, even from the most grueling Brazilian jiu jitsu practice.'

Goggins and Matten hired 37 members to KX Gym in London to check the diet on a broader scale, of whom 15 were overweight. All had performed a small amount of exercise; none had raised it, and some have even continued to do less. And the findings were impressive in just one week, even with the calorie restriction: the test subjects lost an average of 3 kg of fat but placed on about 0.8 kg of muscle. With a standard diet that reduces calories in a week by the same amount, you'd expect a maximum loss of 1 kg.

Why are there no Sirt supps?

It's the obvious question: if sirtuins are so game-changing, why aren't pharmaceutical companies rushing and supplementing to distill them into pill form? Short answer: because the process by which they work is still not fully understood, which means that the body will not automatically consume supplies as well as the natural forms.

Goggins and Matten point to resveratrol as the reference. "In addition form it is partially absorbed by the body, but its bioavailability (how much the body can use) is at least six times higher in its natural food matrix of red wine. They believe it is better to ingest a wide range of these nutrients in the form of natural wholefoods, where they coexist with the hundreds of other natural bioactive plant chemicals that act

147

synergistically to improve our wellbeing. "In other words: eat better, rather than just popping up a pill.

Fast and furious?

This aspect of the Sirt Diet of course has detractors howling. Many point to the fact that the diet relies on calorie restriction at least in the initial stages, and that weight loss above 1 kg per week is unsafe or impossible, according to previous experience. It's a valid concern: in most calorie-restricted diets, early weight loss tends to come from calorie exhaustion and decreased water-bloating, and–as recent research on contestants on TV's The Biggest Loser suggests–actually rationing yourself every day can slow your metabolism to a near-permanent crawl, as well as interfering with your body's levels of "hunger hormone" ghrelin, leaving you permanently hunted.

Yet, address Goggins and Matten, that is not what Sirt is doing. Indeed, the diet mimics certain features of fasting, and the benefits of calorie restriction tend to be turbo-charging within the first seven days of the full diet Sirtfoods. But this is a bit more complicated than just starving yourself for improvements in the short term. How does that work, then? Okay, first, recognizing the "pain" part of the equation is vitally important. "Everybody wants a little tension in their life," Goggins says. "We build stress on the body each time we exercise, which can be a good thing or a bad thing. There is a tendency to always train harder, to try harder, but this carries the risk of building up chronic stress which carries the risk of burnout and a weakened immune system.

The flipside: You can improve your body's ability to cope by exposing your body to low-grade sources of stress. "The reactions to plant stress are much more complex than ours," Goggins says. "Think of it: if we are hungry and thirsty we can go in search of food and drink; too hot —we need shade; we can escape under attack. By comparison, plants are stagnant, and must tolerate all the severity of these risks and physiological pressures. As a result, over the past billion years they have built a highly sophisticated stress-response system that humbles[humans] by creating a vast collection of natural plant chemicals– called polyphenols–that helps them to adapt to and adjust successfully to their environment. We also consume these polyphenol nutrients when we consume these plants which activate our own innate pathways of stress-response. Here we are talking about exactly the same directions that turn on fasting and exercise-the sirtuins.

According to Goggins, polyphenols are the only thing that the typical American diet has enough of, and the much-lauded Mediterranean diet lacks almost all its value when deprived of them. Polyphenols have a host of weight-management effects through Sirtfoods, including promoting white adipose tissue (the usually bad stuff) to imitate brown adipose tissue (the "healthy" fat that helps generate body heat).

149

These also assist with issues of completeness by increasing the response of your body to the satiety hormone leptin.

"Because of their ability to turn on the same positive changes in our cells as would be seen during starvation, such as fat burning, these natural plant compounds are now considered' calorie restriction mimetic'," Goggins says. "The game-changing consequences. When we are presented with more sophisticated signaling compounds than we are generating ourselves, the effects are comparable to anything that we alone can achieve.

The real health foods

There's definitely more to Sirt than to body structure, though. Further statistically controlled trials on single Sirtfoods have shown promising results outside of the Goggins and Matten studies. For example, in October 2015, researchers at New York's Columbia University discovered that drinking water with a gram of cocoa–especially rich in sirtuin activator epicatechin–dissolved therein led to improved memory in 19 middle-aged subjects.

Scientists at Monash University in Melbourne reported in November of the same year that, when patients in the early stages of type 2

150

diabetes applied one gram of turmeric a day to their diets, their working memory strengthened. There's some support for diabetics that sirtuin activation increases the amount of insulin that can be secreted and can make it work more effectively. In the skeleton, the sirtuins stimulate osteoblast growth and regeneration, a type of cell responsible for building new bone.

When more research is done, the next big thing for Sirt will be in its connection to leucine, the strongest muscle-builder among the branched-chain amino acids (BCAAs). Leucine is a key protein synthesis regulator and stimulates a protein known as mTOR (though you don't have to think about that to grasp the next bit).

"Leucine is a double edge sword," Goggins explains. "It's an acceleration for muscle growth, but if you don't have the internal equipment to support it, the motor can blow." In principle, getting a more syrtfood-heavy diet might increase the amount of protein the body will assimilate effectively, placing the old suggestion "20-30 g a sitting" squarely into the past.

All that, of course, needs more research. Thirty-seven participants in one gym are not much of a sample size, and other studies have been done on the impact of sirtuins on animals or human cells—neither are they expected to accurately reflect what is going on inside the body. But for all the skepticism of the diet's more extreme statements, following some variant of the Sirt Diet, it's hard to see what you stand to lose. Even if you put aside the calorie-restricted version of the diet and jump straight into "maintenance" mode, you will eat a huge variety of foods defined as essential in the so-called Blue Zones, world places like Sardinia and Okinawa where people live longer, healthier lives.

"I don't like the term diet but it's lifestyle-like food as opposed to some quick-fix action," Donald says. "It's about living well, in fact. Yet given the popularity of green juice drinks, the overall philosophy is about adding balanced whole natural ingredients rather than' superfood' deification. "Or, to put it another way: you're unlikely to become less nutritious by having more spinach, almonds, walnuts, yet red wine into your diet. Even if you're not a UFC fighter or a supermodel.

Foods that can increase certain protein levels are known as sirt foods. Some of the best-known sirtfoods are below:

Turmeric

Buckwheat

Onion

Walnuts

Coffee

Strawberries

Blueberries

Medjool dates

Dark chocolates

Kale

Red wine

Soy

Matcha green tea

Extra virgin olive oil.

You should eat these foods as part of the sirtfood diet, and limit the calorie intake. A mixture of these two stimulates the body into developing higher sirtuin levels.

The diet was created by two celebrity nutritionists who work at a UK private gym. We say that adopting this diet would lead to rapid weight loss, while retaining muscle mass as well as providing disease protection.

How to follow Sirtfood diet for weight loss?

The diet has two stages, each lasting 3 weeks. You can then include as many sirtfoods in your diet as you want in your meals. Studies say this diet can help you shed about 3 kilograms in a week's time.

If you see the sirtfood page, they have foods that can be found easily in your kitchen. You should know how to prepare sirtfood green juice before going ahead with the way you practice the sirtfood diet.

Kale, arugula, parsley, celery, ginger, green apple, lemon and green matcha tea are all required. All ingredients except matcha tea and lemon juice. Water the lemon with your palm and add it to the water of green tea powder.

Step one of the sirtfood diet is 7 days in length. You'll need to limit the calories to 1,000 calories for the first 3 days. You'll need 3 green juices and one meal to drink. Sirtfood omelet, stir-fry shrimp and buckwheat rotis are just a few things that you can consider.

You will increase the calorie intake by up to 1,500 calories over the next 4 days of phase one. You can have two green juices and two or more sirtfood-rich meals in one day. The very flexible sirtfood can be used to prepare meals.

The second phase of the sirtfood diet lasts 2 weeks. This process is also called sirtfood diet maintenance phase. In this process you are to slowly lose weight. There are no limitations on calories you need to meet in this process. You can have three full meals in one day, plus one glass of green juice.

You should replicate the two steps again in case you want to, to achieve the desired weight. In reality, the diet can be your lifestyle, rather than a one-time diet that you took for weight loss.

Is Sirtfood diet sustainable?

Sirtfood's antioxidant and anti-inflammatory properties will provide potential health benefits for you. But, because of the calorie-restrictive nature of the diet, you're at risk of nutritional deficiencies. It is not recommended to eat 1000 calories in one day without adult supervision.

Top tips:

Be Kind to Yourself-Sirtfood Diet Tips

If you want to eat something delicious, you should eat two squares of dark chocolate (15-20 g) each day, containing at least 85% cocoa. And although in the first week you'll have to opt out, you should drink a small glass of red wine with two to three meals a week during phase two.

What to Drink-Sirtfood Diet Tips

You should drink as much liquid as you like throughout the first process-as long as it is non-calorific as plain water, green tea and black coffee. A splash of tea or coffee in the milk is ok. Try adding strawberries, lime, basil or lemon to water for a sirtfood flavor.

Tip: Adding some lemon juice to green tea ensures you can absorb more nutrients that cause sirtuin and burn even more fat.

Meal Ideas-Sirtfood Diet Tips

Consider soy yogurt with mixed berries, sliced walnuts and dark chocolate for tea, or for something savory, a bacon-packed omelette, red chicory, and parsley.

The sirtfood salad is perfect for lunch-but if you want any carbohydrates, a whole meal pitta with turkey, cheese or hummus is balanced and satisfying.

It doesn't have to be boring at dinner time either: stir-fried prawns with kale and buckwheat noodles are a great evening meal. However, believe it or not, if it's made the sirtfood way pizza is still on the menu.

Chapter 8

How To Do The Sirtfood Plan

You may have heard about the Sirtfood Program before-especially after singer Adele was confirmed to have lost 50lbs following the program-but do you know what it really is?

The eating plan describes the twenty ingredients that turn on your so-called' skinny genes' to increase your metabolism and energy levels. This simply stipulates you can lose 7lbs in 7 days...

The eating plan will alter the way you eat well. It may sound like a name that is not user friendly, but it's one that you're going to hear about a lot.

Because the' Sirt' is slang for the sirtuin genes in Sirtfoods, a group of genes called the' skinny genes' that function, frankly, like magic.

Eating these foods, say the plan's founders, nutritionists Aidan Goggins and Glen Matten, turns on these genes, and "imitates the effects of calorie restriction, diet, and exercise." It triggers a recycling process in the body, "which cleans out the cellular waste and garbage that accumulates over time and induces ill health and vitality loss.

Such foods contain high levels of plant chemicals called polyphenols, which are thought to turn on the genes of Sirtuin and thus activate their super-healthy effects.

Red wine, cocoa (dark chocolate!), and coffee are among the top 20 Sirtfoods. Buckwheat is the biggest carb on the list, and that was the popularity of the first book–The Sirtfood Diet–when it was released last year, that it was sold out by health food shops, and buckwheat noodle maker Clearspring had to double its production.

Want To Lose Inches? There's The Weight Loss Plan

How to do it: Two or three days, you drink three Sirtfood Green Juices a day, and have two Sirtfood meal and 85 percent Dark Chocolate 15-20 g

Lindt Excellence. Day 4 to 7, two greens a day, two Sirtfood meals and one chocolate snack.

Conclusion

The plan will detoxify your body for seven days and then you'll need to keep eating sirt foods to see weight coming off, or you'll get it all back. This diet is not very healthy because, for most people, you're eating two of your meals, which isn't sustainable in the long term. It is a diet for those who are following a fantasy, and ready to pay for it. It in no way resembles usual feeding and I assume it is unhealthy. It is a very intense stuff. The green juice revolts, and I poured some down the sink. I hated tossing all the harvested fibers onto the compost fire, feeling that I would have enjoyed eating all the juice ingredients in their entire state and that it was better anyway.

Due to the high cost of exotic foods and the amount of time you'll spend juicing and cooking your meals, this diet will be incredibly hard to follow for many reasons. If you don't like matcha or kale then you'll find this diet very hard to follow as many of the Sirt Food Diet recipes contain both of these ingredients. Most people just flat out hated the way the drinks smelled, and couldn't even bother with the diet. The Sirt Diet program includes two phases:

Phase 1: This process will limit you to 1,000 calories a day for a week, and two of your meals will be green drinks rich in Sirt Foods such as lettuce, celery, parsley, green tea and lemon. Even rich in Sirt foods like beef, chicken, spinach, or buckwheat noodles you can have one meal per day.

Phase 2: You are permitted to increase the caloric intake to 1,500 calories during this process and you are still consuming the two green drinks, but you are now permitted to add another meal to the day, allowing two meals and two beverages. This phase can last up to 14 days.

This diet is certainly not for everyone, and it requires a lot of funds and energy to get through the meal preparation. The book includes several recipes about halfway through your reading, but many of the ingredients are so special that consumers found it hard to find them at the grocery store, as well as the tastes were so different in the beginning. Generally, this diet is backed by science, as many case studies have been shown, but for the average person the possibility of seeing results from this diet alone is a long shot.

Lightning Source UK Ltd.
Milton Keynes UK
UKHW021334290421
382828UK00005B/16